I0790456

BUMPISM

For The Second pregnancy and beyond.

ANNA ERIKSSON

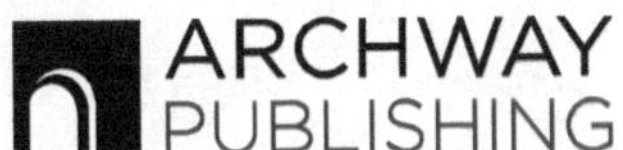

Archway Publishing books may be ordered
through booksellers or by contacting:

Archway Publishing
1663 Liberty Drive
Bloomington, IN 47403
www.archwaypublishing.com
844-669-3957

ISBN: 978-1-6657-2966-6 (sc)
ISBN: 978-1-6657-2967-3 (e)

Library of Congress Control Number: 2022916698

Print information available on the last page.

Archway Publishing rev. date: 09/22/2022

CONTENTS

THE FOREWORD

Over the last three decades, (*yes I
know it seems like a really long time),*
Pregnancy has gone from something you
only whispered about behind your hand,
To now having a sort of pregnancy culture.
Everything is about the Bump!

Women no longer have to feel that pregnancy is
a medical condition, or a shameful but necessary
fact of life, because we've been made to feel for
the last 300 years that it's an affliction. But now
pregnancy is back to being a celebration of life,
with the modern generation all shouting "it's all
about the bump!" and that is how pregnancy
culture has evolved into something bigger then
the natural process of creating life. We have these
before things now called a "gender reveal party"…
What happened to a good ol' fashion baby shower?
Now in the late 80s finding out the gender of
the baby was a little difficult, ultrasounds were

not that high tech yet, And lot of time you had to wait. My parents had to wait, well that and I kept rolling over. So they had to really wait 9 1/2 months to find out what I was.

But more about the pregnancy culture... Only just 9 years ago when I was pregnant with my first child, little had changed about the social views of pregnancy as it was from the decade before. Not much has changed in the way baby gear, except for now designer baby gear is a thing, You could pick up, for a whopping $25, three onesies that said air Jordan or Pollo or Nike, Heck I'm pretty sure Coco Chanel has a baby onesie collection now as well, But that aside the evolution of pregnancy and pregnancy culture has changed quite a bit. 9 years ago people were more afraid of natural birth and it was a push from all sides for medication interventions, and if you wanted to do things naturally with no medication they thought you were crazy. Now lets fast forward 9 years you have a whole subculture to pregnancy culture that want you to stay away from the medication, and stay away from medical intervention, it's turning the tide saying that "If you're seeking help you're obviously doing it wrong" when in fact you're just trying to deliver your child safely. Many advancements and achievements have been made in the last 9 years.

A great advancement from a female doctor that did this study showing the women of African American descent were at the greatest risk for one of the more deadly pregnancy complications called preeclampsia and her research lead to show that preeclampsia is preventable with diet changes and the addition of a specific easy to get over- the-counter medication and we didn't even know that 9 years ago.
The culture of pregnancy has advanced significantly. In some ways to excess, but in other ways very positive. I hope you enjoy the book and I hope it brings you laughter, a better understanding, and the community connection to entire network of women who have gone through this journey you are now going through. The same Joy, excitement, rage *(Believe me you will have rage toward the end like you won't believe it'll make the Incredible Hulk look like a giant pansy.)* There will be tears and embracing moments, But you're pregnant, what might have been embarrassing before is totally excusable because… you're growing a human.
So relax and sit back put your feet up, because believe me kankles are just terribly uncomfortable and we deserve the rest.

And enjoy!

FIRST TRIMESTER

I found myself pregnant again, eight and half years later. I discovered after doing research that there were no books about the second pregnancy that gave me helpful and emotional understanding. No two pregnancies are the same so I thought why not write one that includes the stuff you know and the stuff you didn't expect, or you just plain forgot.

Week 1

Now this book is about your second pregnancy not your first.
Your first pregnancy everything goes according to the rules… mostly. Every pregnancy after, the rules do not apply. It's like this is the week your body prepares for ovulation and that happens

in the first 24hrs after you peak. As I explain to people that are TTC *(trying to conceive)* the way you tell if you've ovulated you notice during testing is that you'll see *(high peak high)* the day after the peak the second high is ovulation and you have 24 hours to do that baby dance.

Week 2

Post Baby dance, now for many of you baby number two probably wasn't planned, many of you do not remember the last time you did this. But trust me that egg is already snuggling in for its nine months nap.

Week 3

Now is the time you think you're going crazy, your sense of smell will suddenly be heightened and that hidden pair gym socks, that is under the couch, from three weeks ago will rear it's ugly head and you'll be able to pinpoint it's location. You also might be slightly crankier than usual thinking *"Oh it must be PMS."* But once you find the socks, you may feel little sick and you quickly put them in the laundry and close the door and hope you don't have to go in there until it airs out.

Week 4

Now the PMS symptoms really seem to be at threat level yellow. Your boobs will hurt and much more than usual, you'll be cranky, you'll also start craving things. Some women even experience implantation bleeding, some do not. And all you're thinking in the back your mind is *"This period is going to be AWFUL.".* But something feels off. If in 10-12 more weeks you find out you're having a girl there is a good chance you might be puking at this point and be thinking *"that seafood salad must have been spoiled, I better throw that out even though I just bought yesterday".* But if you're having a boy you could just be excessively cranky and the smell of some things may be a huge turnoff, where as before they were huge turn on, like your husband cologne or the smell of fried food.

Week 5

Yep it's late! You're seemingly regular scheduled visit from aunt flow didn't come, now you're considering maybe *"I'm just stressed out and waiting another day or two and your period will come."* But then again the symptoms are little bit telltale and you're wondering… *"when was the last time I had sex?"* Because you're busy, you have another child, and you're standing there in your bathroom counting on your fingers going *"umm"* or you're looking through your phone and you realize *"Oh wow!That was almost 4 weeks ago maybe I should just test and be sure because it's probably nothing."* And then… That nothing, is a something with a PLUS sign.

Breaking the news is always fun.

Week 6

Because this is your second time around the block with pregnancy things will happen faster, your bump will pop faster, the bad hormone responses like nausea, exhaustion, drooling… you might have never drooled during your first pregnancy when you're taking a nap, but now you will suddenly wake up with a pool of drool on your pillow. You will have new cravings, different cravings.

Week 7

Now the fun begins you may have not needed to pee as often with your first pregnancy, now you're running to the bathroom more often, you will just lay down for the night and in 30

minutes you'll have to pee… Again! If you've
already started having morning sickness there
is another condition that comes with morning
sickness which is an extreme form of morning
sickness. Some women do get it. It's actually
more common with your second pregnancy
than your first and some women never get
it at all. *HEG (Hyperemesis Gravidarum)

*A severe type of nausea and vomiting during preg-
nancy. Rarely, morning sickness is so severe that
it's classified as Hyperemesis Gravidarum.

Symptoms include severe nausea and feeling faint
or dizzy when standing. It can also cause persistent
vomiting, which can lead to dehydration.

This condition can require hospitalization and treatment with IV fluids and anti-nausea medications.

This was not in any pregnancy book I first read. I
did research of my own when it happened to me.

Week 8

Now comes the confirmation appointment,
you get to see the baby for the first time and
the little heartbeat no matter how many times
you have an ultrasound, It's still exciting. You

might be also investing in cases of ginger ale, your partner may be excited because the Tata fairy has arrived again. But they learned the first time you can look, but… no touchy!

This is also the time you decide if this is the doctor you want as your doctor for delivery, or do you want someone else, and or you might need a high risk specialist. I know, that last one sounds scary, but they handle things that a normal OBGYN can't or might not feel comfortable with doing. Some, but not all qualifying factors are… If you are 16 and pregnant, or 35, and pregnant. Those are cases that may or may not need specialist care. You could have gestational diabetes, be a type 1 or type 2 diabetic pre pregnancy, have high blood pressure, low BMI or high BMI, hormonal imbalances that lead to miscarriages, etc. There are many factors, but now is a good time to start looking for a doctor, if you want to change.

Week 9

Since this is your second pregnancy, this week since your uterus has already stretched once before, now it'll stretch faster and that small slight bump will be a lot more prominent. If you invested in maternity clothes when you were at

15 weeks the first time, now you might want to start looking at maternity clothes at 10 weeks or at least the stretchy yoga pants the dressy looking ones because you're start filling out faster.

Week 10

10 weeks down, 30 to go!
Its all about the small victories.
If you haven't already noticed the bowels will either slow down or speed up at this point, the vaginal discharge will start to change. It becomes thicker and more like gelatin and less like water or egg whites. Also for some lucky women your morning sickness is waning,
But for some it may continue.
My doctor recommended B6 vitamins for my morning sickness and it might be something you discuss with your ObGyN before testing.

Week 11

If you are over 29 like I was or this
is baby number 2, 3 or more,
you might find that your previous discreet bump,
is bumping out more partly from gas and bloating,
but partly from your womb being familiar
with the great stretch its about to perform.

But also with being older when you have another child, you tend to need more naps! Fatigue is very common in the first and third trimester, napping was my favorite part of the first trimester.

Week 12

The bump has shifted north and is really not hiding itself well. Which means you won't need to pee as much. But if this is baby number 2 or beyond, then the bladder still has trauma from the first pregnancy which means… "you sneeze, laugh, or cough … you will pee or as I call it squirtle." Because it's not enough urine to empty your bladder, but it's enough to warrant you using a protective liner.
You may or may not be less tired, that depends if you have other small children. Food or life smells might not be so abrasive, a lot of books and or people say eat healthy, now that you can eat, but you just finish puking for 3 months, eat slowly but enjoy yourself.

Week 13

As previously mentioned, some symptoms disappear, sometimes they don't. Around this week you're supposed to get the "pregnancy

sex drive", there is a good chance that the
baby will throw a monkey wrench into
the works and there will be no hanky-
panky until the babies is late or born.
This is about the time most people are starting
plan their "gender reveal party"… others have
invested in the home blood kit that allows you
to find out the gender. I don't recommend the
blood kits. If you have infertility conditions that
are hormone based, the test will be wrong and
you have wasted $112 that you can't get back.
Something I used, that I'm sure other people
would not agree with was the Chinese
Gender Prediction chart. It actually works.
I'm not sure why it works, it might have
something to do with astronomy and other
mathematical algorithms that were used
hundreds of years ago, but it was the only
thing that was accurate long before I had
the sonogram to determine the gender.
This is also the time when you want to start
looking at maternity clothes. It might have been
a while since you bought them or it's your first
time buying them, a lot of those clothes are
super cute but they're also super expensive.

I discovered five things that are comfortable
that you can wear again. Now I'm a plus size
woman and I found a lot of my shorts, (not

from maternity shoppes) but from plus size
clothing stores like Torrid, Romans etc.
A lot of those pieces I still use today
I altered them to fit now.
And I added alterations that I
could let out or take in.
A flannel shirt can be an amazing accessory.
Maternity Leggins at Walmart, that are just cotton
are extremely affordable and you will go through
multiple pairs and they fold up nicely so that
you can keep a pair in the car for "accidents",
Not like automobile accidents but more of "oh
no I just vomited all over myself while driving".
I always kept a spare shirt, pair Leggings,
and pair of underwear with a panty
liner in my car at all times.

The other thing you're going to need is proper
shoes. One thing I noticed everyone was
wearing the same sandals from target. But
these sandals actually provide zero support
and will give you a lot of back pain.
I ended up getting slip on sneakers from Torrid.
And later I bought orthopedic shoes, my
husband helped me put on and I could
slip on myself from orthofeet.com.

My last big suggestion for the end of the
first trimester is start looking into maternity
bras that also become nursing bras.

Many great brands like Kindred Bravely.
Were amazing for a maternity bra, but
after I started pumping and breast-
feeding they were too small for me.

Another good bra to look into is dairy fairy.
Dairy fairy is very good at accommodating
different sizes and it actually has an opening
so you can pump and not have to unhook
your bra and it's hands-free but you can also
pump and Breast feed at the same time.
The only con about it was after I stopped
breast feeding it was too big.

Remember we get bigger, faster the
second pregnancy and beyond, its
always good to be comfortable.

Remember : big is not a bad word.
Big hearts give more love.

** for some this might be the end of your
first trimester for others you might have
one more week in the first trimester.
It depends on how the numbers add up.

❧

THE SECOND TRIMESTER

Welcome to the second trimester for many
of us we're getting a spring back in our
step, we're going to start nesting again.
But if you have a younger child in
the home already you might be
wondering why did I do this again.
I just got back to sleeping. But
it's worth it in the end.
By now you're probably wondering
why I haven't really mention much
about the baby because there's literally
hundreds of books that are just about
the baby growing inside your womb,
And they'll grow the same way. But there
are no books about what happens to
us the second time around, and that's
what this is about, it's about us.

Week 14

By this week "hiding" the pregnancy news will be difficult because you're definitely showing. Another thing that pops up that you didn't notice the first time is round ligament pain, now you might have experienced this much later in your first pregnancy. But the ligaments are stretching from the hormone "Relaxin" *(yes that's what it's really called).* This time it will happen faster, suddenly you'll have pain you didn't have before it's kind of like twisting your ankle and getting shocked at the same time.*(Sounds pleasant, right?)* There's some prenatal yoga stretching and other stretching techniques you can do to lessen the pain that comes with this and makes you more limber. Some Tylenol and nap also helped me *always talk to your doctor first before using any medication.

Week 15

By this time hopefully you should be able to eat real food, and maybe catch a glimpse of what the gender is. A lot of us say *"okay this pregnancy is going to be the one, Eat all the healthy stuff, and exercise often…"* yeah it doesn't happen or it does. But in reality some of those healthy choices are great for one gender, but they're not for the other.

If you want to double up on the healthy portions
of a plant- based proteins like tofu, that's great
if you're having a girl, too much of a soy based
diet or vegetarian base diet when carrying a boy
can be detrimental to testosterone development.

Being mindful of what you eat can also impacts
the chances of gestational diabetes, the
chances of high blood pressure development,
and the chances of unsafe weight gain.
Not to say that you might still be
carrying the weight from your previous
pregnancy, which happens.
Try just being the best you!

Think of this week as the steppingstone
to the rest of the pregnancy.
Something other books don't talk about is,
that when you're high risk all you think about
is getting to the point where everything is
going okay! I will say from experience, when
you're pregnant there is no point where it all
becomes okay until you're holding that baby.
But don't allow your stress and your fear to
be all- consuming try to talk to your partner,
or talk to other women who have been in
the same situation as you. Also make sure
that your physician understands about
being high-risk. As I mentioned previously

when you're thinking about finding a doctor
you might need high-risk a doctor.

**Also Little Side Note.* While you start down the
journey of being able to eat again, You might
start getting heartburn this week too, and you
have never had heartburn likes this before,
But you'll never have heartburn like this again.
Unless… You decide to have another baby.
Because pregnancy heartburn is like Olympic
size heartburn. It's trained all your life just to be
this miserable when you're pregnant because
it knows there's nothing you can take to make
it better, so it's just going to be a beast!

Week 16

Something else that can also happen this week
is dizziness, fatigue, and lightheadedness.
Dizziness can be the result of a few things,
But I always found it occurs when I stand up
too quickly. And because you have blood flow
going to different places now, dizziness will
occur more often, especially with your second
pregnancy. Lightheadedness can occur when
standing as well as When you're sitting down.
I keep Snacks in my purse for when I get
lightheaded that are healthier than a candy
bar. But also The Atkins protein bars, the

good ones like…cookies and cream or
blueberry yogurt or strawberry. You can also
keep regular granola bars in your purse.
Fortunately there is nothing that helps with
the fatigue, during my first pregnancy, The
second trimester was everything they promise
you it will be. But when I was pregnant the
second time… It was not that awesome,
it was also the start of summertime and I
was tired all the time. Not solely because I
was pregnant, But because it was hot and I
was bigger this time. Pregnancy dresses are
your friends, not necessarily ones that are
gathered and fitted on the sides but the ones
that are maxi dresses knee length or longer.

This is the week they also recommend
that you see a dentist.
The one thing that you don't realize is that
pregnancy is more than just growing a
human, it also takes nutrients from other
parts of the body… that even a prenatal
vitamin cannot completely replace.

And sometimes no matter how much
we brush, floss, or mouthwash our
teeth and gums will suffer.
Bleeding gums are very common. With all
of your blood vessels opening up, more
blood flow is showing up in other places.

It wouldn't be that uncommon for
you to have a bit of blood when you
brush your teeth while pregnant.

You'll also notice an increase in vaginal discharge
something you might not of noticed before
but that's okay because if you followed my
advice in the beginning you invested in some
cotton panties and some panty liners. But if
you're concerned that there might be a leak, I
definitely suggest looking into something like
always discrete pads they really do lock away
the fluid for the sneeze-n-pee moments.

Week 18

Stretch marks!
Now you may have developed many
of these from the first pregnancy,
But you might not develop that many this time
around because you already stretched once.
It doesn't mean that you shouldn't do
proper moisturizing care of the bump.

Week 19

You're almost there you're five months at this
point, but also something creeps up that you

may not have had the first time… I know I had it the first time and the second time… is the Leg Cramps! I'm not talking like *"oh I didn't stretch before went for a run"*, I'm talking about Full on, wake you up in the middle of the night muscle wrenching cramps, it's like someone took your kneecap from behind your knee and just torqued your calf muscle. Now something that works to prevent it, has to do with how hydrated you are and where your electrolytes are.

I started keeping Gatorade by the bedside, you can do Gatorade zero if you're a gestational diabetic because they use Splenda but I would definitely double check with my ObGyn because Splenda does cause high blood pressure and if you're also being treated for high blood pressure, that can be counterproductive.

Other things that are a little more natural, that are good to keep handy as well is coconut water. Coconut water is naturally balanced with electrolytes. I drank a lot of it because I didn't want to run the risk with the Gatorade zero and it has a good flavor, find one you like the best. Also Body Armor is amazing because it's a natural version of Gatorade, it has a pleasant flavor, it's made with electrolyte components that come from the coconut water, and they make one that's called "lyte" that is made with stevia.

Week 20

Now with this week you are literally halfway there
40 divided by half equals 20.
If you were just starting to show durning the first
pregnancy, you're really showing now, and a little
person inside is really starting to do "The Cha-
Cha" or they could be practicing some kickboxing,
While aiming at your ribs or your hip. The best
part is what you eat, they're going to eat. If
you want the baby to have a taste for healthy
things or have diverse taste this is the time to
eat healthy, because when I was pregnant with
my first child I did not eat the healthiest food.
My 1st child loves healthy foods anyway, my
second pregnancy I ate lot of healthy foods, and
diverse foods. My babies enjoys things like Middle
Eastern food, Indian food, fish, strong flavored
foods. The food choices I made had an impact
on the likes and dislikes of the children, outside
of the womb, when they started eating. They say
that when you eat spicy food it will make the baby
kick because they'll taste the spice in the amniotic
fluid. But before you *"cancel those hot wings,"* it's
not so much that it bothers them and yes it does
make them kick, but they'll develop a taste for
it when they're born and when they get older.
A lot of pregnancy books are going to tell you
try to make healthy choices instead of giving

into your cravings. If you have a craving and
it's something that is safe indulge! I mean
don't sit there and eat 5 gallons of ice cream
every night, But if you want a cupcake eat
the cupcake! If you're on a restricted diet,
that you think your only options is to eat
vegetables and chicken, Then your dietitian
is wrong and hates life. There are so many
things you can do and it will be extremely
interesting. There's a lot of healthy options on
a Chinese menu, there's a lot of options at any
restaurant or in any cookbook that are not
loaded with bad things for your blood sugar.
But you can definitely eat what you want
and not feel bad about it, If you do it within
the right perimeter, there are so many
things you can eat, but yet so many things
you need to watch out for in foods.

Sometimes we crave things that we would never
normally eat when not pregnant, but they could
be harmful when we do eat them. I personally
craved Paté, and there was a place back in the
day that I could get Paté where I used to live.
This French restaurant offered goose Paté,
but it was not foie gras, it was goose liver, but
from geese that were fed things like kelp and
seaweed, and in a humane way. It completely
changes the flavor, and made it healthier it had a

richness… yumm! Liver is not safe when you're pregnant. My cousin she craved oysters so badly when she was pregnant, and oysters are not safe. The Mercury content is way too high. There are many options when it comes to fulfilling your craving safely and within reason.

Week 21

If anxiety is something you're experiencing this week, you are not alone! One in five pregnant women start to experience anxiety around this week because it's sinking in again *"Oh no, we're doing this again"* Some women only get pregnancy anxiety the first time. But being a second time mom and depending on the how far apart your kids are in age, you still might get that little bit of anxiety and a little bit of frustration because you're not just carrying another child you're also taking care of one that might be younger 2-6 years of age or might be a little bit older 6 and up. Sometimes some of the stress and anxiety can come from outside of pregnancy, like every day life. I know this is when some of the pregnancy rationale comes in to play. Your husband might notice and not react or he might walk on the egg shells till that baby is born. Or you might notice that things that didn't bother you now really bother you. The way someone snores, the way someone pops their gum, and it's not you, it's not them, it's the hormones.

Your firstborn might be amazing, an angel and you're thinking "*This was a good idea, that we did this again.*"
But then you hear the horror stories.... "*Oh my god! What if the second one is nothing like the first one?*" Relax kids are not carbon copies, each child has an individual personality. It's going be okay. Deep breathing exercises really can help with the anxiety if you feel you're having a panic attack I do the gratitude spacing technique.

That technique starts with closing your eyes taking three deep breaths in and out make sure you can hear yourself breathing out. Then you describe the first five things that you can see when you open your eyes, and describe them out loud. Then you think about the five things that you that you can hear, and you described them out loud.
Keep breathing!
Then you describe five things that you're grateful for and they can be the most mundane things like
"*I didn't Pee myself today. Or had my favorite yogurt for breakfast.*" Nothing is too small

or too big to be grateful for especially
when you're doing this exercise.
And if you have to cry because everything
is just overwhelming… you cry, because
that's your right, you're pregnant, no one
should ever tell you you can't cry.

Week 22

If you ever wonder why you waddle like a duck
when you're pregnant? Part of it has to do with
your hips separating… we will get to that later.
The other reason is because you're duck footed.
Some people have narrow feet and they might get
a little wider, But then they go back, So they don't
actually change. And then some of us our feet
change a whole size and a half! Staying that way
even after the babies born. Your feet will swell.
The swelling will go down, but the bone, tendon,
and cartilage adjustment does not change or go
back. Everything stretches and flattens out to
balance, changing your gates so you can support
the belly in front of you while you're walking. A
lot of women go for the comfortable shoes, you
can just slip on. But if you have extremely high
arches like I do they will be uncomfortable. I
ordered a lot of my shoes from torrid. Torrid has
these adorable little slip on sneakers in many

styles and patterns and they were perfect. I didn't have to bend over to tie them, because they're was wee bit of elastic to hold them on your foot and they were super comfortable.

Week 23

Somethings that starts to appear this week, especially if you are blessed with a darker complexion! You develop a dark line from just at the top of your pubic bone all the way up to the bottom of your sternum, it almost looks like you're pregnant belly has a baby zipper that's under your skin. I know that sounds super sci-fi, but I promise you it's perfectly natural. I did not have one my first pregnancy I was incredibly pale,(*"I still am incredibly pale"*) but some women Will have more prominent line it's called a Dark Line or in medical terms Linea Nigra.

Something else also start appearing around this time is called the Mask of Pregnancy. Some women that are blessed with a darker complexion will see a darkening of the skin around the forehead, cheeks, eyes, and it looks like you're wearing a mask. This will go away after the babies born sometimes it takes 2 to 3 weeks. Also something else that happens around this time some women will start to develop

other skin conditions. If you're suffering from
vitamin deficiency, or a blood sugar imbalance
due to just gestational diabetes you can develop
strange hyper pigmentation of the skin or
your skin will change in texture around your
mouth and chin area. It's kind of dry and scaly
and it really won't go away, But then suddenly
four weeks after the babies born everything is
back to normal like it was in the beginning. It's
something to definitely ask your doctor about.

Another thing to start trying is meditation I
don't suggest trying to sit with your legs crossed.
Because sometimes once you get into that
position, you can't get back out again without
help especially when you're pregnant. Let's sit
comfortably on the couch put your feet up or lay
down in bed listen to some really good music
it helps you get into that meditative mood.
I don't recommend anything that's on
a specific hz that is for deep healing.
Just because its good for you, some
vibrations are not good for the baby.
Its a good time to get a foot massage.
If your spouse won't do it, find somewhere that
specializes in foot massage and not pedicures.
The harmful toxins in the air that come with nail
salons is not safe for pregnant women, unless
you know one that is extremely well ventilated.

Week 24

Now the stuff you may not have noticed
before is starting to ramp up during
this pregnancy, drumroll please....
Red and hot hands and feet, carpal tunnel, skin
tags, hair and nail growth, extra saliva, blurry
vision or change in current vision, reflexes
and timing, funny tastes, being overheated.
Yeah that's a lot but it's only for the next few
months and sometimes 2 to 4 weeks postpartum.

<u>Let's start with Red and hot hands and feet</u>

Your blood is circulating at a faster rate, its
all because you're growing a human! Your
extremities will start to generate a lot of heat or
collect the extra fluid from the body and start
swelling. (I had horribly swollen feet and hands
when I was pregnant the second time. And my
husband gave me wonderful foot massages to
push the fluid out by using an ancient Chinese
medicine technique. But elevating your feet
above your heart like sitting in a recliner, or
laying down and putting a pillow under your feet
works just as well for alleviating the swelling.
Now as for the red and hot... I usually,... even
to this day postpartum, will stick my hands,
before bed in cold water from the bathroom

tap and it completely takes away the hot feeling that I still get. When your hands and feet are hot, it feels like the rest of your body is just overheating, and you can't properly cool yourself. Your hypothalamus is working overtime trying to regulate your body temperature, Because you're growing human, But if you're older, you've already done some other damage to your body, in some way, shape, or form. Not just from growing the first human. You will be overheated more easily then you were the first time, especially if you're last trimester is in the summer, no room will be cold enough. And your family will say, they're freezing.

Carpal tunnel

Carpal tunnel is an odd little condition that you get when you use your hands and wrists the most when you were working. If you were a cashier or you work with computers you'll develop that one way or another *"I on the other hand developed it from writing all these years "(teehee)* and also working with computers and working retail in college. But it never really bothered me as much as it did with my second pregnancy. I was in horrible pain, I had to sleep with my arms crossed over my chest like Dracula in a coffin. I'm pretty sure that's why he slept with his hands over his chest because his carpal tunnel was so tenacious, even being undead. Now towards the end of your pregnancy they will offer you something. My doctor offered cortisone shots, to handle the pain. The shot isn't really worth it. If the person doing the injection isn't perfect with their aim, they may hit the bone, you will have more pain than you started with. It also can come with the numbness. And the numbness starts in your fingertips, and works its way down. By the time the numbness set in for me, I was about eight months pregnant and it made diabetic testing easier, because I couldn't feel myself poking my finger. But it made buttoning my shirt, holding my cell phone, or trying to use the breast pump a lot harder because I didn't have enough feeling to feel what I was gripping. This part of it can take up to four weeks postpartum for it to completely go away, and you have the feeling back again sometimes longer than 4 weeks when it was completely gone.

Skin tags

Skin tags are growths that develop on the surface of the skin, because of either a virus or your skin cells are multiplying at such a fast rate. Because you're growing human

the additional cells just accumulate, and
sometimes it happen because of friction.
If you don't like them and you're just repulsed,
you can contact the dermatologist postpartum
and it's very simple to have them removed,
it's usually done same day in office.

Hair and Nail Growth

If you ever had okay hair and okay
nails, wait till you get pregnant.
You don't really notice that the first time
because you're just so focused on the bump,
That you never look at yourself and suddenly
this time you do, and you realize *"Oh wait, my
hair looks gorgeous, I look like I could be in one
of the shampoo ads. And my nails are growing
like crazy and they're hard! I don't need acrylic."*
Part of that is the vitamins. If you continue
taking the vitamins postpartum as well, It helps
with the healing processes as well as, help you
restore what your body lost during pregnancy.

Extra saliva

Now this is where it gets tricky, saliva production
increases at the beginning of the pregnancy.
You will notice that when you're napping you

might start to drool that's pretty common,
unfortunately the minor amount of drooling
doesn't stop after the baby is born it kind of
stays with you. But at this point you'll notice
a significant uptick in saliva that you might
not have notice the first time or remember.
Because of the significant amount that
started developing this week, I do suggest
you start sleeping on your side with your
head supported. Many times I woke up in the
middle of the night because I rolled over or
something, and woke up choking on my saliva.
I did not sleep well from this point until the
end of my pregnancy, because I was either
in pain, or suffocating myself on drool.
Try wrapping your pillow in a bath towel,
that way you're not changing your pillowcase
every or washing and drying it single night.

Blurry vision or change in current vision, Reflexes and Response time

Sometimes you're lucky you have 20/20 vision all
the time. But with pregnancy you might develop
vision issues that are only linked to pregnancy,
and go away after the babies born. Not right
away usually a couple weeks postpartum.
Like me you might have astigmatism. Pregnancy
actually changed my prescription so significantly,

I didn't bother getting new glasses, I just didn't
wear them, I also *"much to my own frustration,"*
but for my own safety at the six months mark
of the pregnancy, I stop driving myself places.
I let my husband do all the driving, which for
someone that is independent its very difficult
to let go. When your vision starts to get fuzzy,
your reflexes do too, and you need your reflexes
and response time when you're driving.
Some doctors recommend you go see
an eye doctor during your pregnancy to
make sure that everything is okay.

Funny taste

Funny taste in your mouth, This one I didn't
really experience the way most people do,
they say that they, *"taste something metallic
or coppery."* Some of that metallic,
copper taste actually comes from when you're
pregnant, your gums will bleed. Other times
your mouth might be really clean but you just
taste something off. It's a very strange anomaly
sometimes it does happen to people, it's definitely
something you want to bring up to your doctor
if you noticed a reoccurring taste that is not
normal because it might be something else or it
might be nothing. But let the doctor or midwife
tell you its nothing, Don't just write it off.

Now that we finished our list of symptoms
here is a non- symptom topic.
Something you should consider at this point is…
If your doctor has more than one doctor in the
practice try to meet with all those doctors so in
case of an emergency, if your doctor is out of
town, when the time comes, at least you know
who the other doctors are in the practice.

Week 25

I discovered this when asking other pregnant
women some pregnant women get UTIs, and
will get them the entire pregnancy. UTI is the
anagram for Urinary Track Infection. One of my
close friends had kidney infections her whole
pregnancy, off and on with her second child. This
isn't in most pregnancy books, if it is, it's like a
cliff note or margin notes in the back of the book.
It's not something to disregard, it does
happen in many cases; Especially with second
pregnancies, it might even go unnoticed until
your next appointment because you don't have
any pain, or you can still empty your bladder,
possibly the kidneys might be acting up.
Adding to your water intake is also excellent. Keep
a gallon of water in the refrigerator. And cold
water is excellent during the summer months for

some women drinking plain water can get boring, I use some of the true lemon packets or the true orange to boost the flavors, but not adding sugar.

At this point during your pregnancy it wouldn't be uncommon for your pubic bone, and your hips two separate again like they did once before. Sometimes it goes unnoticed in the first pregnancy, it just happens and *"Oh well, you were walking normal but now you're waddling."* But when its your second pregnancy or beyond, it can happen a lot earlier and it's not unnoticed. It can feel like you got kicked in the butt and it hurts, You stand up wondering like *"Oh my god"* and it's kind of a sudden *"Pop"!* None of the other books ever said that you would actually feel this happen, But apparently you can and I wasn't the only one. Don't forget something at this point that is incredibly uncomfortable, *"Yes, we always know our feet, our legs, our fingers, will swell because they are our furthest extremities."* But you can also (*much to my displeasure as I found out from my doctor),* Because our belly is more extended this time, Because of the previous pregnancies you can also accumulate fluid in your torso, around the womb, under your skin like you would your fingers, hands, or feet and it makes everything tight. And terribly uncomfortable and to top it all off, you can barely breathe. If you start to discover an unnecessary tightness in the area where your Bump is definitely tell your doctor. Because that is their job, to answer your billions of questions, that those other books never told you about.

Week 26

This week the count begins. Everything you eat is going to start to add towards the end total of yours and the baby's weight. How fast you and the Baby gain is not so much quantity, its quality. Making good healthy choices doesn't have to be boring, nasty, or gag worthy. That's why there's going to be a section of the book that is nothing but food choices and recipes.

Some women experience round ligament pain in the very beginning, slightly In the middle, and in the very end of pregnancy. I had it the whole time with my second pregnancy, it's going to ramp itself up this week because now everything is out side of the *"containment zone"* let's call it that. You should be really bumping out now. You should really have a full bump, now that your ligaments are receiving more of the hormone chemical Relaxin *(I know it sounds like I made that up, but I guarantee you that is what it's actually called, I'm pretty sure a guy came up with it, because that word sound like a hair care product.)*

Week 27

Now starts the last week of the second trimester you're in the homestretch, although you probably feel like you're stretched beyond capacity. If you're at this point you're probably sitting there going, *"Why did I think this was a good idea to do this again?"* If your babies are two years apart, You should still have the majority of the products you used the first time like a breast pump, If your babies were further apart like mine were, and you have health insurance you can use the program AeroFlow. They will get you your compression socks, your bellyband, your postpartum compression trousers, and your breast pump. If you have had a problem with breast-feeding in the past or with pumping, the pump you use makes all the difference. I didn't know this until my second child and the lactation consultant said that I needed a medical grade pump, Medela is a brand of medical grade pump, and your insurance should cover it especially with a doctors note. You won't receive your breast pump until about three weeks before delivery, But at least you are all set. Now you can buy a breast pump from the store or rent one from the specialty pharmacy, I still recommend Medela. Other brands are terribly popular like Elvie, because you're wearing them inside your bra and they're wire free. These are ok too, but not if you have a problem with *"the let down"* during pumping.

When you're this pregnant, you definitely need to be prepared for heat rash. Getting overheated is very easy in the summer, I would almost prefer being this pregnant in the winter because you're kind of like your own built-in furnace, protected from the cold. Many years ago they said *"Pregnant women can catch a chill faster than someone who wasn't pregnant."* That's not 100% true. It can't be cold enough when you're pregnant because you're always overheated.

Thats not to say you shouldn't take proper care during the winter, its just easier to overheat. And you don't realize how overheated you are until you go for your postnatal visit and you realize that the waiting room is freezing, Because you're no longer pregnant and overheated. Now you know what your husband was complaining about the whole time. If you're also on a lot of support hormones for being pregnant you will experience a very strange shift after the baby is born, and your

body has to readjust without those extra
hormones. You'll think you're going through
menopause. Especially if you're older then
30 when you have your 2nd second child.
I know we talked about swelling in the last
part of the chapter, But its a greater reality
when you're older that you have a chance of
developing preeclampsia especially during
the second pregnancy. Some cravings you'll
have over and over again like salty chips,
extra crispy bacon, a whole watermelon, all
of those have really high amounts of sodium
either artificially added or naturally existing
And can cause swelling and edema very quickly.

You may also be experiencing more bloating gas
this time then you did with the first pregnancy.
Check with your doctor to see if it's okay to
take Simethicone, also known as Gas x.
This is also the week that heartburn is going to
rear its ugly head, and you'll have that until the
end. There are two types of heartburn, One is
like liquid fire shooting up your esophagus like
red hot lava. The other is an alkaline type of
heartburn not many people get, But it is truly
miserable, because there isn't a way to truly
neutralize it without making it worse. It feels
like ice shooting up your throat, and it makes
your stomach burn and swell. And makes eating

anything miserable. Ice cream? *"Yeah, that's a great idea, you're never going to get heartburn." "Oh, A glass of milk?" "Yeah, to give you more heartburn."* Nothing will take care of or prevent it. When you have that type of heartburn you have to decide *"Is that food going to be worth it?"* Then decide on maybe something a little more wholesome so when you do suffer at least you know the baby got enough sustenance, even if you're to be miserable.

CHAPTER 3

THE THIRD TRIMESTER

Week 28

Well were in the home stretch!
Now the days of having all that energy,
and that extra room to stuff with
food are Gone with the Wind…

Now you just want to nap, and you're
back to the needing a nap regularly.

If you have smaller children when they nap, you nap just like when their a baby, get as much sleep as you can and now. Try to fit your household tasks in during the burst of energy for the day, if you have any. Bending over is probably gone by the way the dodo till after the baby is born. Now is a good time to invest in one of those reach and grab things on a stick so you can pick stuff up.

Lifting your arms above your center of
gravity too high, is also dangerous.
Its dangerous for a few reasons, now this one
is an old wives tale, But it is actually true, and
I do know someone it has happened to. The
umbilical cord can move when you stretch and
reach above your head too much, and can get
draped around the baby's neck. That is one of the
many ways babies are born with the umbilical
cord around their necks. If you need to reach
something up high or put something up high,
Use your grabbing stick thing, do not climb on
things. The bigger you get the more unstable
you will get, and judging the distance between
the next step down, and the floor might be
different, and you can fall. It's best to be careful!

Okay now that I'm done scaring the
crap out of you. Lets start with what
you should be feeling this week, That
they might not have told you about.
Sciatica is a huge possibility, it's like someone
threw a dart at your butt, and instead of hitting
the "bull's-eye" they hit the nerve that runs
down off your spine, and down your leg. It starts
with a sharp pain that shoots downward into
your leg and you're just like *"Oh snap."* when it
hits, you'll probably say some swear words you
never thought you were able to say, and you

hope to gosh your little one didn't hear you.
Because you know they're going repeat It.
Stretching, wearing proper shoes,
and proper posture will also help
with this when you're walking.

If you feel like you're getting a cold, but you have
no other symptoms besides a stuffy nose. Its
from the extra mucus production, and regular
swelling that happens during pregnancy.

Week 29

Alright it looks like we're down to the 11th hour,
we've got 11 weeks to go, starting today.
Remember when you thought pregnancy
looked cute, but now its not feeling so cute!
Everything now is just uncomfortable!
Now I do recommend looking into photographing
every week and keeping a picture in your
phone. Or if you are into scrapbooking,
make a pregnancy scrapbook just for you.

Varicose veins may not happen during
your first pregnancy, they may happen
this time, And they don't go away.
You can have corrective surgery if you really
care about how they look, But the surgery
is more painful then you could imagine.

Some women get hemorrhoids, it's just a fact. The extra pressure on your intestines creates the possibility of constipation. It seems 9 out of 10 women will suffer from constipation that is a fact, But you don't have to if you eat fiber and drink water. Little bit a lemon in water before bed at night (I know that sounds crazy) but it actually works. And it might give you a little heartburn. If you drink warm water and lemon first thing in the morning instead of at night you will still have a bowel movement. Some lucky people have IBS-D which is <u>Irritable Bowel Syndrome with Diarrhea.</u> Being pregnant gives us more of a regular cycle of bowel movement, or it aggravates the diarrhea symptom of our IBS-D, and you can't run to the bathroom fast enough. The outcome of this effect really is dependent on the individual. I know when I say *"fiber"* you're probably thinking *"Oh, I need to use Metamucil or eat vegetables raw or just tons of vegetables... blah".* No, just green apples or just regular apples, like Honeycrisp! Apples have an amazing amount of fiber in them that is digestive fiber, and it can stave off hunger, it can regulate your blood sugar, it can help with digesting meals so you're getting the full saturation of your nutrients. Apple also contain Malic Acid which is great for fibromyalgia pain.

Broccoli is also pretty fibrous, but Broccoli will also give you a ton of gas… it's not worth it. Cabbage although a little gassy is very fibrous, it's a good green, collard greens when cooked properly are extremely good for you, and excellent for getting the gut moving.

Week 30

The baby makes their way into their final position. If you're lucky that means the babies get to be in the head down position, and that's a good position to be in. Because then it's only their feet that are going to be kicking you in the stomach, ribs, and in the lungs it almost feel like at times. But if you're like me you get a snuggle baby, and they want be as close to your heart as possible and they will stay in the breech position till the end, and then suddenly decided turnaround if they still have room to. Once I hit this point I could not sleep comfortably, I was more tired when I woke up, then when I went to bed. I would come home and take naps or take naps in the car to and from appointments. My husband did most of the driving to appointments. I was too big to reach the steering wheel and I'm short,

"Put all that together and it just wasn't possible."
Getting one of those pregnancy pillows might be
a good idea, or it might be a big waste of money.
I will say the first pregnancy, I didn't need to
sleep with pillow between my knees, actually
found it to be incredibly uncomfortable. The
second pregnancy on the other hand, with it
being hot all summer long I didn't want anything
touching me, I found that putting my leg up
on something was a lot more comfortable.
At this point all of those horrible early pregnancy
symptoms can come back. Your breasts
will be larger, and tender. As if they weren't
tender the first time the Tata fairy showed
up. Now they're just sensitive and irritated,
and you're irritated because you have too
big boobs sitting on an even bigger belly.
You might have a repeat visitation of morning
sickness, except instead of the morning…, it's
all day long and it can be at anytime. Around
this time I had no control over when I was
going to throw up it would literally happened
within seconds. That's why some unfortunate
cashier at Walmart will never be the same.
He said "hold on let me go check" and I said
"I'm sorry I can't…" and before I could finish
my sentence he was covered from head to
mid torso in vomit. Because for some reason
I was blessed with a high-capacity spray, and

that was due to the extra pressure from the baby's head being under my stomach, and I think the muscles were just well toned from throwing up throughout this pregnancy.

Don't worry if the baby is sitting breech durning this week. The baby still has 10 weeks to turn over, and put their butt up and head down. And don't let the doctors and the medical staff make it sound like breech is a bad thing it's just different. Unless there is cause to worry. It just means things my have to go differently, it's not the end of the world.

Week 31

If you're still feeling up to a little bit of hanky-panky at this point with your partner, I suggest you try some of the positions you've always wanted to try that doesn't put you on your back, or have you laying on your tummy. Orgasms are good for you because they help you relax but more importantly it gives you a break from the extra stress that comes from just being pregnant.

If you feel like you're shorter on breath, or walking, being pregnant, and breathing all at the same time is just way too difficult when you're in the grocery store, Do not feel ashamed to use

one of those motor carts. Some of those motor
carts are actually slightly tweaked in the motor
and it will go faster than they should and you
can be a crazy pregnant lady flying through the
store. Make your partner do all the walking, don't
stress yourself out or overheat more than you
have to. The baby is getting plenty of oxygen via
the placenta so while you're gasping for breath,
they're okay. You will feel a decrease in fetal
movement, But if you feel no fetal movement
for more than a couple hours don't be afraid
to call the doctor. Especially if you get up, you
move around, you shine a light on your tummy,
you fidget a little bit, and you feel nothing
definitely call the doctor or go to the hospital.
It doesn't matter what time of the day or night,
they always have people on call. This is their
job, It's what you're paying them for anyway.
At this point till the end, you'll be making
quite a few trips to the doctors office or
Labor and delivery department of the
hospital where you plan to deliver.

Planning a direct route or alternate routes and
driving them regularly will help you become
familiar with those routes. It is extremely
important when the moment comes and it's time
to deliver. Because a tree might fall, there might
be a thunderstorm that night, there could be

traffic, you have no accounting or control over the idiots on the road or nature for that matter.

Week 32

I've mentioned before about writing down a *"birthing plan"* This would be a good time to start writing down the things you want. I'm going to include a link in the back of the book you can source to find different types of birth plans. Now remember this is just an outline because sometimes things don't always go according to "plan".
If you went to birthing classes the first time you might not have to go again. There are some really great ones that you can watch the videos on YouTube, all of the classes I took were off of YouTube, because there weren't any classes in my area.

Lightning crotch is also something that can start happening this week. It's like you'll be sitting there and suddenly you'll get this shocking electrical feeling in your cervix, like one of those buzzer rings that when you shake someone's hand gives you a buzz. That has to do with a few things. It stops just as quickly as it started. And can just take you off your guard. Lighting Crotch usually happens within 4 to 6 weeks before delivery.

It's kind of like the baby doing a practice round
of dropping down near the birth canal and
putting extra weight on the nerves down there
and then pulling back up again and waiting.

Something else super delightful that
happened around this time for me was, my
right rib near the bottom of my rib cage
became dislocated. And it required seeing a
chiropractor that felt comfortable with trying
to relocate the rib, Because of the amount
of pain and pressure I was going through,
I couldn't sit comfortably without the pain,
I couldn't stand walk, or breathe without
the pain, and it went from dull to sharp.

Week 33

Hello Braxton Hicks Contractions!
These practice contractions in your first
pregnancy, they had you running to the
hospital every five minutes. But there is
a slight difference between real and BH,
If you feel like you're being squeezed
from the sides that's Braxton Hicks,
If you feel pressure from the top of your
uterus and the top of your bump that's the
real deal, You definitely want to call your
doctor about those and start keeping track.

Some women who have slight infertility
issues or severe infertility issues will have
start/ stop labor from now until the end.
I started having the start/stop labor around
this time and it would be horrible, until I got
to the hospital and then everything would
just stop, and I wouldn't have dilated at all.

I also had gastritis.
Which sounds awful and it is, but it's
basically the Stomach lining has become
so irritated that it swells up and creates
more pressure in its confined area. It's
kind of like your stomach is chafing.

Something to look out for in these weeks. That
is not in any of the books, I actually had to
Google this and read it in an old textbook.
You want to start making sure if you feel pain
in your right side, in the right part of your back,
and the right front call the doctor immediately.
This could be HELLP syndrome. Your body is
starting to shutdown because of your Liver.
That is super scary and if you had high blood
pressure in your last pregnancy, the odds
might be elevated this time around too.

It's something to be aware of but don't
stress out before you have to.

This is also the time to start talking to your
partner about being your labor advocate. If
your partner is not an outspoken person, or
not a go-to person and they don't have a strong
personality, they might not have it in them to be
your advocate, and advocate for your choices,
your health, and your rights as a patient and
that's okay. You might have a family member or
a friend that feels comfortable doing this for you.
You can also hire a person called a Doula that will
be that advocate for you. My husband was 100%
my back up advocate, because I could definitely
advocate for myself. If you had a bad experience
with your first pregnancy, because people
wouldn't listen to you, you need to stand up for
yourself this is your body, this is your baby, now
is the time to get it right and heal from the past.
But this is the week to sit down and
have these discussions with your
labor team. Form a real plan.
Because everything will start
snowball from here.

Week 34

At this point I was just waiting for them to say
"Okay, the time has come for getting that baby out."

There are a few tests that happened that
are pretty regular and your partner isn't
there for them. Because usually room is
small, and there's other women in there too.
For privacy reasons they tell the husbands
they have to wait in the waiting room.
Man does that seem to make them
mad. My husband was furious
because its not explained well.
But all of us gals are sitting there with our
bellies out and our feet up, some women
are from cultures where only a woman's
husband can see her tummy exposed or she
can be seen by other women. So its why its
a *"No man zone."* Unless you are a doctor.
But it's a very important test, and you get
to bond with the other moms who are
due around the same time as you and
you get to share your experiences.
And it's kind of what inspired me
to write this book actually!
Other than an entire list of quirky little
quotes about my daily happenings.

NST TEST (Non Stress Test)

You get to sit and relax in the chair with your
legs up, that's the best part! They put one
monitor on one side and Another monitor

on the other side to monitor fetal heart rate and to see if the baby's heart rate changes because of agitation or movement I never quite got, if they wanted the baby to be agitated or if the baby is to not be agitated. But at the end of it you get to have another ultrasound and you get to see the baby again. When you have a high-risk pregnancy you get to have a lot of ultrasounds. When you don't have a high-risk pregnancy you get fewer ultrasounds, but it is always exciting to get another ultrasound.

Sometimes you have to repeat this test multiple times in a week or over the course of the next few weeks. But you're there for at least 45 minutes, and that is 45 minutes in a nice cold room, that is the most important part in the summertime. Your legs are up and no one is bothering you. If you want to fall asleep and snore… they even put a blanket on you so you're comfortable. And you get to talk to the other women, if they want to talk to you, if you're not a social person just read a book. I am a social person and I talked to the other women I learned about them and their cultures. It was a lot of fun. Some of us ended up bonding and when we would see each other in the waiting room, or leaving, or when we were running in and out of labor and delivery every other night we would Say *"Hey, how are you doing ?" "Is it go time?"* And then I came to find out a lot of the husbands while sitting grumble to each other while sitting in that extremely cold waiting room. Saying "Why can't we go? Whats going on?"

After the stress test you go get an ultrasound, and you have to be squeezed in between the other schedule ultrasounds, so they don't really have time to run to the front office to grab your partner. You just get to show them a cool picture when you leave after your three-minute ultrasound.

Week 35

Only five weeks to go till 40
weeks, Till the due date.
And Sometimes you feel like you're 17
months pregnant. It's been forever, you can't
remember the last time you actually felt good.
You will do stuff, and say stuff, and act
irrationally, and people look at you like you're
crazy. I know there were many times my
husband went and said to my mom *"Please
tell me this is will be over soon."* And my mom
says *"It gets worse after she has the baby."* And
it is worse after. I just feel so bad for him, I
have almost no memory of being like that.

But it's all pregnancy hormones, you're going into a survival mode. Mostly because you're so pregnant, the world starts to bother you. And that is part of our deepest primal instinct to protect our offspring. More about that later.
If you haven't packed your bags yet. Now's the time to start. Just to have in the car so it's ready to go. And when the *"Go Time"* happens you're not running around going *"Where's my bag"*.
Or have it packed and by the front door so that you can just grab it as you walk out the door.
They usually tell you, you don't have to bring your pregnancy book. My book is not some heavy chunk of reading material, so yes totally slip it into your bag, because there're sections in here you might need or I hope you don't need. But I believe in being prepared for everything and anything. So prepared that I made my husband learn how to deliver a baby in an emergency. Because we live far back in the country it takes 30 minutes to get to town and it takes us 45 minutes to get to the hospital. So he needed to be prepared. I Already knew how to do it but he needed to learn in case I couldn't reach down there and deliver the baby myself.

Some babies… Second and third and fourth and more pregnancies come when they're ready, and sometimes that's early.

Some schools of medicine originally
thought that pregnancy was completed
at 35 weeks and you only needed the
last five weeks to fatten the baby up.
Now they're discovering that going the
full 40 is better for lung development.

Some babies come out when they're ready
one of my friends went into labor with
her second child at 38 weeks. The baby
was considered two weeks premature.
But the baby was perfectly healthy.
It's all about you and your baby and your body.

Week 36

According to traditional pregnancy books,
about your first pregnancy. You'll start
waddling at this point. Lets be serious we're
veterans at this, this is our second or beyond
pregnancy we started waddling weeks ago.

You will have continual round
ligament pain until the end.

But you will notice something this week that
happens for some women it didn't happen for me
it's called a lightening. The baby will drop, from

where they are sitting on your stomach, kicking you
in the lungs to dropping down into the pelvic area.
That will take some pressure off of your
stomach and your lungs, you will be able to
breathe a little bit better, But your gate will
be severely off, you'll be a little more clumsy.
You will look like John Wayne getting off a
horse that he was riding for seven days.

Take your time, don't go around sharp
corners quickly. Everything can wait.
You'll get there when you get there.

If you're feeling a lot of pelvic pressure at
this point it is possible that your cervix
is starting to stretch a little bit and you
may even dilate a whole centimeter.
When you feel a strong amount of pressure in
your pelvis and standing or sitting isn't really
helping, hold on to the counter, or the side of
the couch, and plant your feet flat, or stand on
the balls of your feet if you can, and squat down
pulling your pelvis, but more importantly pulling
your vagina to the ground and you'll feel that
gravitational pull, then when you stand back up
the pressure will be gone. Gravity is your friend.

Being comfortable at this point is the
most important thing. If you can get a
couple extra hours of relaxation in sitting
on the couch, lots of pillows propping
you up and creating extra support, and
you end up sleeping there, just sleep.

Week 37

If you're at the point where you're worried
that the baby will never come and you
will be pregnant forever. There's plenty of
things you can do. A lot of times they say
go for a walk. At this point you're starting
to get annoyed with your doctor, when they
give you stupid suggestion like that.
I will tell you a secret, if you are very active,
like I was with my first pregnancy and you
walk everywhere anyway, and you do a lot of
exercise. Walking isn't going to do anything.
But one thing I did notice was three days
leading up to when I actually went into labor
every time I was up walking around for long
periods of time I got really excruciating back
pain that would make me sit down or I would
get pain in the top and the sides of my womb.
We didn't know at the time that those were
premature labor pains that were starting

and stopping. If I had continued with the
walking and then started doing the squatting,
I would've actually gone into labor three days
earlier. Listen to your body and pay attention
to the signs it's giving you that it's ready.

Sex can also speed things along, part of the
female orgasm is actually a uterine contractions.
If you're on an activity restrictions because
of a problem with the placenta which they
should have detected at some point during
one of your many ultrasounds. I would say
to avoid sex because it's rigorous and the
cramping can actually cause a problem.

Now this suggestion falls into the realm of
homeopathic medicine, but it's true! if you
haven't started dilating or had a bloody show.
Then it's been known that the hormones in
semen can cause the cervix to start to relax and
dilate but the same amino can also be found
in evening Primrose oil capsules and many
midwives have used that over the centuries
when you run late to start natural Labor. You
can ask your physician or midwife about that.

Don't look at this as a waiting game.

Weeks 38-40

These weeks can all look the same.
You might not make it to 40 weeks that
baby might show up at week 39.
If you haven't decided on a baby name
yet now is the time to really give it some
consideration. You might be really set on
calling your kid Rupert. But then when you
see the baby he's actually a Connor.
In my family we believe the baby knows it's
name, before it's born. You might not know its
name until they tell it to you and this comes
from a deep interconnection the mother has
with the baby and it's something you feel.
But you might also want to have a few girl
names picked out. Sometimes babies might
appear one gender in the womb and when
they're born they might have different parts!

You might've painted that entire nursery
for a Bonnie or Rebecca. And now you
got to paint it for an Anakin or Jared.

Also don't be ashamed to use family names
if you have some awesome family names.
I specifically didn't use family names,
except for my first child's middle name
and that was to carry on the tradition of
using a different version of William.

But his first name... 100% reflected that his mom was part of a very important fandom. *"And he shall be the only child with his name."* If that doesn't give you a hint what it is, I can't give you more hints or I might have to pay someone.

Just be prepared.

When packing your bag these are the important things you need above all else. Get disposable underwear. Birth is messy, it is not dignified in anyway, you're going to have a lot of afterbirth that's going to be coming out, don't waste your cute $40 underwear on that. Buy disposable underwear I recommend the Always brand because they have a better odor shield. Afterbirth has a very distinct bloody smell. Invest in good smelling butt wipes, bird baths are a thing if you had a c-section.

Don't pack your breast pump because the hospital will have one. Many hospitals actually offer the Medela breast pump and they have a lactation specialist there to help you with getting the baby to latch on, and all that important stuff. Pack yourself a couple of the men's flannel shirts. Your partner can wear them as well and you can wear them. They are great when you're breast-feeding, Because They're

warm and they're soft but you can also
cover yourself, whatever you want.
If you're plus size gal like me a lot of the
cute maternity nightgowns didn't fit me.
Instead, I ordered a lot of nightgowns with
the button-down front that you see in the
grandma catalogs, like Dr. Leonard or Carol
Wright, and they're much cheaper or the
same price, and offered better coverage.

Make sure you pack socks that are slip
resistant and comfortable. I recommended
diabetic socks because they'll stretch
you probably still have kankles.
A nursing bra.
Your bra size will go up significantly once
you start pumping buying a bra in the next
couple cup sizes up is a good idea.

If you're larger in the cup size before
pumping then DD cup you might need a
different type of bra that has more support.
These comes from a different company
than Amazon or Kindred Bravely.
Some bras offer the Multi option where you
can pump and feed it the same time, This is a
good idea. Your breasts will actually start to let
milk down when you're feeding on the opposite
breast. So hook up your pump to the free breast.

Lactation pads are important! You can get
reusable ones for home. I don't recommend
those for the hospital. I recommend getting
disposable ones because you won't have
anywhere to run and wash them, and
the reusable ones are kind of pricey.

If after the baby shower, you don't have
tons of outfits and tons of diapers now's the
time to make sure you have your extras.

Back up formula.
Do your research if you're going from
breast to formula. For whatever reason.
Don't go straight for the standard blue label
formula those can actually be very harsh
and super caustic on the babies gut.
The gentle Versions of those or the comfort
versions of those are what you want to
try, If you have to convert to formula.
It's good to just have a can on reserve just in case.

If you got a bunch of different brands of diaper,
first use all the samples you got, and see which
ones you like. some diapers actually have
a great absorbency compared to others or if
one baby did well with one brand the second
baby might not do well with the same brand.

Make sure you include three outfits for the baby. Include in the diaper bag, two newborn sized, and two 0-3 month sized outfits. My reason for this is if the baby's projected pre birth weight and length is 7lbs and 20in. Sometimes when the baby actually arrives, the baby is 10 lbs and 19in long, or 12 pounds and 26 inches long. The cute newborn outfit isn't going fit and you need a 0-3 or 3-6mos sizes.

CHAPTER 4

THE END GAME

Okay the day has come! We're counting our labor pains, we're timing the contractions, it's all ready to go. But… What is our end game?

The end game is doing what you have to do to make sure you and this baby come home safely.

I mentioned birth plans before and it's a good *"floor plan"* for how you want things to go. But sometimes things don't go according to plan.

We have put some wear and tear on our body between the first baby and this baby. We might be older, or we are over 35, or we develop some of those and pregnancy conditions that put us at a higher risk. Making sure your doctor is on board with this birth plan is a good starting point. If your partner has decided to be your backup advocate, Make sure they understand what their job is, that everything is executed according to your wishes, But also in the best health, and safety interests of you and the baby. If that means that your labor nurse is not doing her job, by ignoring you or being passive aggressive about your pain or experiences, It's their job as your advocate to say *"hey what are you doing, my wife is in pain or something is wrong and you haven't come back in an (blank amount of time)"*, its ok to ask for a charge nurse or a nurse manager. It's not unreasonable.

Home birth

If you're opting for a home birth you don't have to pack your bags, you don't have to go anywhere, you just have to prepare your space and Call your midwife, and to prepare for the realities of the home birth. That Include minimal medical intervention, without outside interference. What that means is, if something goes wrong, (which sometimes it does.)

You have to call the paramedics and be taken to the hospital to either finish the birthing process or for extra interventions.

It also means that you have complete control over your environment. The lights can be lowered, the lights can be on, you can play music, you have your Doula if you hired one. Hundreds of people for hundreds of years gave birth in homes, because there was nothing else. It was the only option. But if you're a high-risk case and you have preeclampsia, gestational diabetes, advanced maternal age, previous c-sections, previous delivery complications, This is not a safe setting for you.

Birthing centers

Birthing centers are kind a like a doctors office, but they're kind of like your bedroom too. They're set up like a doctors office/bedroom they'll have midwives on staff and a doctor that oversees all of it but they might not be there. They often have a birthing pool. There have been many studies that show a water births although somewhat considered unconventional to some, Can be wonderful for pain relief, if you do not want use painkillers.

Swimming is amazing when you're pregnant,
I can only imagine that feeling of being
weightless in the water, and the flow of the
water really helps with contractions.

Hospital birth

Hospital births have become the most
conventional way to have babies for the last 80
years, especially if you live in an area that had
a hospital. You can have the same noninvasive
experience if you declared it in your birth plan
and you have low risks a pregnancy, Then
you can have a similar experience that you
would have at home, but in a hospital... where
someone else's and clean up all the mess.

You can have the control of pain medication
and there's no shame in asking for medication.
Labor is equal to breaking 20 bones all at
one time men could not handle this,
If men had to have babies we would've
died out a long time ago as a race. As it
was told to my mother by her doctor.

All joking aside, there are many options.

Squatting down every time you feel a contraction
come on, if you didn't have an epidural,
Can speed labor up significantly.

In many countries and cultures throughout the
world today, Women actually practice this as a
means of pain relief during labor and/or delivery,
by bearing down and pulling their birth canal
towards the center of gravity, towards the earth.

When getting into squatting position use the
support of your birthing partner or Doula
And squat down, Bring your birth canal
towards the earth make sure when you squat
down your knees point out like a butterfly and
take a deep breath in and breathe out as you
squat down you'll actually feel gravity pull
the baby down, this can be helpful enough
to allow you to do most of this laboring at
home if you live close to the hospital because
it will speed up labor significantly.

Things to be aware of when you're doing
most of you're laboring at home is the
bloody show! It'll be a little bit of spotting
and usually when that happens, it's right
before the babies about to come.
You need to be heading towards the
hospital before the bloody show starts.

A lot of hospitals want you to labor while laying down that does not help. If they have a problem with you going through labor while standing up, or while squatting, or being able to move around because you have a pre-existing risk condition like preeclampsia, you need to discuss a different birth plan.

Now sometimes we go through all of this beautiful labor for everything to come to a screeching halt. You're fully dilated, everything is ready to go, But The baby stops progressing downward and out. Do Not Freak Out, sometimes this happens, it's important that you and the baby come out of this safely. If they have to do an emergency C-section they will either do a twilight anesthesia, which is a state of asleep but awake or they will do a spinal block. If you've already had an epidural, the C-section is nothing, they just give you extra medication. During an Emergency C-sections you will be awake for, and they'll pull the screen down so you can see the baby when it's born, and it's the longest and shortest 45 minutes of your life. And then they pass the baby to your partner and you get to see that little person and it's amazing.

Sometimes if you're like me, if you have
preeclampsia and you have the high blood
pressure throughout your pregnancy, A vaginal
delivery is not safe. And medical intervention
is your only option. You should never feel
shame, pressure, or let anyone make you feel
badly because, you chose to make sure that
you and your baby came through this safely.
If you're scheduling a C-section,
It's a little bit of a waiting process it's just like
the a regular surgery you can't eat the night
before, I didn't eat the night before all I did
was throw up. I had horrendous heartburn,
I was ready to go, in the morning.

They will play music for you, they will make
you comfortable, I had the most amazing
anesthesiologist he was a true gentleman.
At one point during the procedure I said
"hey I don't feel so good, I feel sick to my
stomach." And he made sure I got the meds
I needed. The meds they give you, in your
spine will make you very nauseous.

The Labor nurse, I was not thrilled
with her but that's who was scheduled
that day so it really didn't matter.
My doctors office had many doctors and I knew
all of them, the one that delivered me that day,
I hadn't met yet! But she is probably my favorite

Doctor out of all of them. Among the regular doctors not the high-risk ones. I still see her postnatal. She gave me answers to questions I couldn't find online or in any books, she explained things to me in a way that didn't make me feel stupid, she was really the best. And when we went for delivery and the baby was out all the additional weight I had packed on very suddenly wasn't actually weight. I had accumulated Extra amniotic fluid!
And once the baby was out I started to cramp, *(which the spinal block did not prevent me from feeling)*, and it started to rapidly dump the fluid out. She had to work very fast to get the placenta out, get that under control, and get everything stuffed back inside and sewn backup in record time.

You actually feel no pain with a spinal block C-section. You feel a lot of disembodied pressure and in cases like mine you will feel cramping. But you feel no actual pain. Your partner might faint, they said that happens at least 12 times a day. My husband actually had to go sit in the corner right before they made the initial cut he was like "I don't feel so good". When I delivered, I was actually three weeks premature, But we had to deliver early because my preeclampsia was getting hard to stabilize.

But our baby was over 9lbs at three weeks premature. Some of that had to do with genetics and gestational diabetes.

Something I want you to remember, and repeat this to yourself, have your partner remind you, even if you hire a Doula have them remind you. Any choice you make that brings the baby into this world safely and you leave the hospital alive, it's because you made a choice. That may not have been your original "plan" but you chose to do what was needed.

Preeclampsia doesn't end when the baby is born many doctors still don't take it seriously, especially in African- American women. I currently follow two stories online where the doctor didn't take it seriously, the hospital didn't take it seriously and the husband advocated and advocated but no one listened.

Making sure you have a good health care team that listens and puts the health and safety of the mother as a top priority is very important.

Good postnatal care is very important.

The nurse you were with during labor
and delivery may not be the nurse
that you have in maternity.
With my first child a lot went wrong. From
beginning to end, At this point. What was
more frustrating was the maternity nurse
I had, hadn't been briefed on the situation
or what was going on, and I was very sad
and very depressed after the birth, because
everything about the birth was extremely
traumatizing and post delivery was as well,
if not more. The nurse was just a bubbling,
happy ray of sunshine, who has that positive
but dismissive reinforcement attitude. And
when I said I was very worried and didn't
know what was going on she said "well at
least you had a baby" I didn't know if she was
bringing her own chip on her shoulder to the
conversation or what. But it greatly annoyed
me and too this day it still annoys me.

My second pregnancy

The whole thing from Delivery to Maternity ward
healed a lot of those wounds for me. Having
a rainbow baby after a very traumatic first
pregnancy and birth made all the difference in
the world. A big part of that is having someone

there to advocate for you. Being educated, prepared and asking tons of questions.

That's why I'm writing this book because I had tons of questions, and I'm a bookworm. But there were no books that even touched on some of the stuff I mention here, or made it emotionally accessible to me, and other women like me.

Postpartum

If you gave birth naturally,
Then there is a possibility that you had an episiotomy or you didn't and you have some vaginal tearing. Because there's no way you squeezed something that big, out of the hole that small, without some damage along the way out. If there wasn't that much damage or tearing… I have questions?!

You'll get this lovely spray bottle that You put warm water in from the tap, and instead of wiping which can rip out your stitches you'll spray after you go to the bathroom. It's actually kind of nice if you did have stitches, after you spray and wash with your spray bottle…, which is called the "postpartum peri bottle" you will have something called derma blast.

It's an amazing you spray analgesic that
makes everything numb for a little bit.

Wearing your disposable underwear is going
to be the best thing in the world if you've just
had an epidural and you're coming down off
it there is a good chance you have a catheter.
And if you have a lot of vaginal bleeding instead
of trying to get the disposable underwear on
your nurse will kindly stick a pad there just
to catch the blood with a few underpads.

If you're epidural has worn off and it's been
the 12 hour. They'll remove the catheter and
you have 12 hours to start going on your
own, drink lots water and eat lots of ice.

And when you go to the bathroom if you are
having a hard time getting the flow to go,
try running water it will make you pee.

If you've had a C-section elective or emergency
you will have a catheter the same rule of going
to the bathroom applies, but when you stand up
to walk for the first time, because they want you
to walk so that you don't get blood clots it will
hurt, it will be uncomfortable, you will look like a
baby pterodactyl taking its first steps outside of
the nest. My husband thought it was the cutest
thing, I flipped him off. Some hospitals have a

postnatal protocol that right after the delivery,
and all the way up until that 24-hour window,
but for the first 12 they'll do it every 30 minutes
to an hour. They'll come and rub your tummy
if you had a C-section they come in and check
the incision to make sure it's still sealed and
you're not gushing blood and you can't feel it.

It is painful! They're rubbing something
that's trying to contract back on itself and if
you gave birth naturally it's not so bad when
you give birth via C-section it's terrible. I
think I drop more f bombs in public then I
usually do, and some those nurses were nice
and I apologized, my one just laughed.

Something else that happens if you
had an epidural or spinal block.

When you're nerve endings start coming back
alive after the meds are starting to wind out of
your system, you will itch like crazy. Everything
itches your skin, your back, your legs, your
face, your arms, it feels like you have millions of
mosquito bites and you can't scratch all at once.

I don't particularly like pain medication,
Because it doesn't actually kill your
pain it just makes it worse.

After the first 24 hours the morphine had come
out of my body from having the spinal block and
I told the nurses I didn't want any narcotics.

One of the doctors from the practice that
I was seeing came in and asked me why,
and I explained that I don't like taking
them and I'm allergic to a lot of them.

Since my blood pressure was stable and my
blood sugar stabilizing they gave me something
I like to call the miracle mix and all of the
excruciating pain I was in from the C- section
went away and was manageable, I could get
up and walk without wanting to faint.

Now I suffered nerve damage as a child that
changed the way I feel pain. What is mild
discomfort for me could be excruciating for you,
what's tolerable pain for me might make you
faint. So I'm not tooting my own horn, I'm just
explaining that everyone feels pain differently.
Narcotics do pass into the breastmilk, if you're
going to breast feed this is something to consider
and it can have a not so great effect on the baby.

Even if they say "trace amounts". A trace is still too much in my opinion, but that's my opinion.

Breast-feeding

If you can get the baby to latch on right away and drink from the breast awesome! Neither of my babies were able to do that. I had a lot of problems with pumping the first time, and that came from the trauma I went through, There was very little good healthcare for pregnant women, where I lived at that time. With my second baby I received so much help and positive reinforcement and those girls worked with me one hundred percent.

All the crazy kinks that came with breast-feeding from *"if you have hormone problems, or you have hormone infertility you're going to need the medical grade pump.*

If you're only able to pump successfully for the first two to four weeks with full milk *"let down"*, and it's an easy process for you but then suddenly everything starts drying up, which can happen. Or even if you make it a few months and you start to dry out. It's okay! That baby got that first week to three weeks of milk from you, that means

that the baby got all your antibodies, and all the
things they need in that first fatty breastmilk.
Called Colostrum.
It was about four weeks when mine started
to dry up. No matter how much I pumped,
no matter if I pumped till I was blue and
bruised, nothing was happening, it was
very little, if anything it was a trickle.
Another thing that happens they don't tell
you about is if you're in the grocery store
and you pump or you breast-feed and you
hear another baby crying… your boobs
are going to hurt and start to leak.
It's a natural, biological response.

It might seem silly to buy two types
of pump but it's really not.
I used a hand pump when I was in the car,
and my husband was driving. because it was
easier than trying to set the whole thing up.
But when I was at home I use the electric pump.
Sometimes first thing in the morning I
would use the hand pump as well because
I didn't have to set the whole thing up.

I felt I got the better output with the hand
pump because I could mimic the motion
the baby makes when they latch on.

Having everything set up when you get
home is the most important thing.

Family always want to do things when a baby
is born, they want to cook for you. If you
have a good relationship with your family and
your friends and they are willing to help out.
Tell them while you're in hospital come over
walk my dogs, tidy up if you want to, Or put a
bunch of meals in the freezer, be my guest.

Something we did was each week Leading up
to delivery, we would buy gift cards to different
restaurants that delivered or something. That
way we had them. If we didn't feel like cooking
we had stuff delivered. I have special dietary
needs but my husband can eat anything. Its
one of the reasons why having people donate
to your cash app instead of bringing some kind
of gluten ridden casserole that you can't eat
because the smallest amount will tear up your
stomach postnatal, Is a better idea. Because a
donation can be made with the same amount
love that they put into that cornbread casserole.

CHAPTER 5

THE PREGNANCY SURVIVAL RECIPES

This might be a bit of a shortlist I'm sorry.
But a lot of stuff I made, I can't
remember all of a sudden but I'll give
you some good jumping off points.

Don't feel so disappointed if they tell you you
have to be on a diabetic diet. If you have a doctor
that basically wants you to eat vegetables and
chicken your whole pregnancy no matter how
much you throw up, find yourself a new doctor
because that's not the doctor for you, they care
about their reputation and not your health. I
actually changed doctors around 22 weeks.

The high-risk specialist I was seeing
was only treating the diabetes and
not treating me like a person.
And the diet was super restrictive and
no matter how much I threw up or I told
him I was gluten sensitive they didn't
care they just kept up my dosage.

So when we found a new doctor and they were
absolutely fabulous they're diabetic specialist told
me, *"I don't care what you eat as long as you eat and
you make good choices."* And then she gave me a
list of how just gestational diabetes is different,
than regular diabetes and how my diet is going
to have to include carbs whereas when I'm not
pregnant it doesn't include as many carbs.

So going from there I created a diet plan
and ate a lot of really healthy food tasted
absolutely amazing and some cheat foods.

I got a lot more variety and a lot more excitement
with my food because a proper adjustment.

These meals I'm including in the recipe section
are Great for just you or the whole family.

But that aside these are great recipes. I made them for my friends who were not pregnant and they just absolutely love them too.

First trimester menu.
These are the foods that I found
easy to keep down that kept me and
the growing baby inside fed.

The smoothies!

Georgia Dreaming

1cup or 8oz the Frozen peaches
6 ounces of dairy milk or dairy alternative
**One scoop of plane-based protein
powder or vanilla whey isolate.

Mean Green Protein

One cup or 8 ounces of fresh spinach
*4 ounces or 1/2 cup heat treated oat.
** one scoop of plan based protein
powder vanilla or whey isolate vanilla
6 ounces of Dairy Milk or dairy alternative
One whole frozen banana or one cup of frozen
banana. (this is good as a smoothie bowl too)
Pinch of cinnamon.

The Tennessean

8 ounces of dairy milk or dairy alternative
6 ounces of frozen banana
One scoop of plant-based vanilla protein
powder or vanilla whey isolate
Two heaping soup spoons full of
your favorite peanut butter.
And a pinch of brown sugar.

All of these smoothies can be turned into
smoothie bowls you just want to make them
a little bit thicker and that can be achieved by
adding a little bit more of the frozen product.

Make Sure that your Protein powder contains stevia
as a sweetener and not Sucralose or aspartame.
If you use unflavored Protein Powder,
honey or Turbinado sugar is a safe
alternative for adding sweetness.

Breakfast

When you're ready for food again, here
are some fun and easy things too try

Many of these recipes can be
made gluten-free or vegan.

Biscuit Buddies

If you're just eating them yourself you probably
need 12 biscuits. Seeing as you're be a little
bit tired I do recommend getting the biscuits
from the freezer, but if you're not tired and
you're in that nesting stage then making
your biscuits from scratch is perfectly fine.

So to make this recipe for yourself and
maybe for other people you're going
to need about 24 biscuits so definitely
get the ones in the freezer section.

24 frozen biscuits unbaked set out to thaw
24 sausage links or vegan sausage links. Pre-cooked
2 cups of cheddar cheese
A Tablespoon of dried chives

Preheat your oven to the recommended
Setting as for what the biscuits recommend.
I recommend using precooked sausage that you
just have to warm because that saves you a step.

Once your biscuits are thawed
Roll them out a little flatter, because they'll still
fluff back up, but you have to stuff them and

get them crimped shut. take one sausage link,
a sprinkle chive and a pinch of cheese probably
a good size pinch, to the center of the flattened
biscuit, fold all the sides together and crimp it
shut so you have like a biscuit log. Place on a
nonstick tray and continue with the rest of your
biscuits till you have no biscuits or sausage left.

Bake for the recommended amount of
time on the biscuit and maybe a minute
longer because you do have stuff inside
that will make moisture, and you want
your dough to be fully baked.

Once these are finished place them in a basket
with a cloth to keep them warm and you can
serve them with honey mustard, Irish mustard,
apple butter or just eat them by themselves.

~ Cauliflower Grits ~

One bag of frozen rice cauliflower
4 ounces of extra sharp shredded cheddar
1 tablespoon of butter
Salt and pepper to taste
2 tablespoons of ranch dressing

I prefer the ranch dressing that comes from the produce section because it has the best natural flavor. Other people prefer the shelf-stable one, it's really your preference. Cook the cauliflower according to the packaging once it's done and you drained away the fluid. Then put it back in the microwave for two minutes so that you can get a little bit more moisture out but then mix in the butter and cheese and the ranch dressing and the spices.

You can and then put a Scrambled
egg on top or some bacon chips.

-The Great Tater Tot Casserole-

One whole bag of any brand of
tater tot that you like I use
Ore-Ida but anything that's about 2lb bag.

8 ounces of cheddar jack or sharp cheddar cheese
*1 pound of smoked sausage, breakfast
sausage, Turkey bacon or vegan sausage.
One of any of those work.

Three green onions stocks

1.5 cups of Sour cream

The large 9in x 13in Glass baking pan,
or better known as the lasagna pan.
Place your chopped green onions, your tater
tots in the first layer and add cheese.
Next, layer on the pre- cooked meat, then onions
and cheese and the last layer of tater tots.
Add the sour cream in a layer
on top of the tater tots.
Then, you guessed it… more Cheese.
Cover with foil.

Bake at 375*F for 30mins. Then remove
the foil and bake an additional 5 mins
to make the cheese bubble.

*If you're using beyond sausage, you are going
to have to sauté it, the same with turkey bacon
and the smoke sausage If you're using breakfast
sausages, I suggest using the pre- cooked
breakfast sausage, its already cooked to the
correct texture, you just have to heat them.

Once its ready, just scoop it out and plate it.
Everyone loves this recipe.

Lunches

I recommend eating a lot of vegetables especially cold ones if you can stomach them, in the summertime when you're probably going to be rounder, and if you're pregnant that time of year you will sweat less. It'll keep your body cooler, and it's easier for your body to process, you're still going to get your carbs with the other stuff *(because you can not practice a keto diet when you're pregnant.)* But you can cut out unnecessary starches which will overheat your body.

Vegetable gumbo was one of my favorites when I was pregnant there's many ways to make gumbo I recommend looking up Justin Wilson.

The diva salad

Two large handfuls of clean baby spinach
2oz Goat cheese crumbs
6oz Grilled chicken
2oz Dried cranberries
2oz Toasted pecans
3oz or 4oz Raspberry vinaigrette
Shake and toss your salad in a container with a lid so that you can evenly coat your salad in dressing and not use so much it covers the salad.

Dill pickle and grilled cheese sandwich

Your choice of bread two slices
One slice of sharp cheddar
And one slice of deli style yellow American
(there is a big difference between name brand
and deli style, deli style has a better taste as
well as less artificial stuff in it) Your choice of
pickle Kosher dill, bread-and-butter I recommend
getting the sandwich stuffers because the
Spears make it awkward. Grill with a little bit
of Irish butter on the outside of your bread
Wait for your cheese to get gooey inside
and then take off heat slice and enjoy or
just enjoy once its cool enough handle.

Salmon bacon what?

1 Butter croissant.
Two or three pieces of smoke salmon
2 tablespoons of softened goat cheese
Black pepper or Tennessee red
chili dust to tolerance.
2 tablespoons butter

Warming butter in a skillet until is clarified.
Put you're smoked salmon in the skillet and
Cook the salmon until it is opaque and no
longer gummy, *(Cold smoked salmon is not*

safe for consumption in its regular state so the method of cooking smoked salmon until it is thoroughly cooked through is the best and safest way to do it if you are craving it and pregnant.)

Once your salmon is completely cooked place it on a paper towel to dry of the excess fat, and then assemble your croissant by spreading your goat cheese on both sides and adding the dusting of pepper or the chili dust and putting your salmon on you can leave it open faced or you can make it into a full sandwich either way.

Fruit and cheese

Thoroughly clean your fruits like pears, grapes, apples, anything you really eat the skin on to make sure you remove any chance of stray bacteria. Choose a nice hard cheese like imported cheddars or Norwegian cheese like ski queen. And make yourself an adult lunchable.

The Pizza Burger

1 frozen turkey burger
1 tostito's pizza party pizza

Cook your burger the whole way through. Cut the
pizza in half, and only bake half if you are cooking
for just you. Bake according to the packaging.

When the pizza is finished cut the half
into half again, so you have 2 squares,
and place the cooked burger on top of one
slice, and top it with the other slice.

This is so good, you family will love it too.

I'm creating categories for you of green
foods, yellow food, and red food

Red foods don't necessarily mean they are
bad for you, but they should be consumed less
frequently then the green or yellow food

Red foods with a ** are an absolute no!

Red foods

Watermelon
Bleached sugars
Bleached flours
Bacon
Most pork products
Bologna

Canned foods with unclear ingredients*
Cool Whip
Tilapia**
Perch**
Grouper**
Snapper**
Raw fish**
Energy drinks

Now I know this list contains items you
should not eat, and some that are okay once
in a while but not the whole pregnancy. Use
good judgment. In the beginning of your
pregnancy you may have had a few energy
drinks before you knew you were pregnant.
**The fish listed all contain parasites. If not
cooked properly, or handled properly, or they're
genetically modified in such a way that they
didn't exist until 10 years ago. some pregnant
women did have reactions to them in the past.

Cool whip is full of chemicals.
White flour and white sugar, or bleached
sugar and flour are made that way by
formaldehyde, which is the same chemical
they use to embalm dead bodies.

* canned foods with unclear ingredients means…
if you can't pronounce it, don't eat it. If it starts

with the words mechanically separated, don't
eat it. It's not's good regularly, I definitely don't
recommend it when you're pregnant. No Raw Fish
just goes without saying, too many risk factors.

There is currently trend about uncured bacon
or uncured meats, I will say if you're going
to eat some of those because you want to
cut down the nitrates make sure they are
thoroughly cooked. Bologna is definitely
something you should maybe indulge in
once if you like it, but not regularly because
many times it's not made with full meat, it's
made with parts. Pork on the other hand,
for heart patients is bad. For a pregnant
woman especially, if you have a problem with
your blood pressure or you have a family
history of blood pressure it's good to avoid it.
Because pork can thicken your blood volume
significantly and in a very short period of time.

Watermelon I know you think think that
would be on the green or yellow list,
But watermelon although healthy
contains a significant amount of sodium
naturally and can cause swelling and
a whole bunch of other problems.

Yellow foods

Organic unbleached sugar and unbleached flour
Natural granola bars
Protein bars Natural
cookies
Natural organic breads
Seltzer water
Naturally sweetened beverages that
do not contain corn syrup
Cream cheese Other types of
melon Half calf coffee
Low sodium or no salt potato chips
Natural peanut butters or nut butter
Boars head deli meat
Gluten-free pizza or regular
Pizza
Pasta

Green foods

Chickpea pasta
green vegetables
red vegetables
grapes
plums
pears
apples
peaches

nectarines
apricots
hard cheeses that are pasteurized
whole-grain breads
heavily seeded breads homemade bread
with unbleached flour pasture raised
butter
cottage cheese
roasted nuts lightly salted
olives
frozen fruit
oatmeal
Fresh prepared chicken breast
Salmon
Low sugar yogurt
Skyr
Natural ice cream

I shopped at Trader Joe's rather a lot when I was
pregnant. Because they had everything I needed
and I can stock my house with all the healthy stuff,
but all the good stuff too, I wasn't giving anything
up for that. I would enjoy things like Oreos but they
did have their own brand which was healthier and
they had a gluten-free brand that wasn't bad either.
I don't recommend it for all of your shopping
because there are cheaper places to buy
meat in a better quantity, but for things like
eggs and frozen food and fresh food and
cereal, chocolate, this is the place I went.

CHAPTER 6

PREGNANCY PSYCHOLOGY

What does this mean?

Well it's something most doctors have tried over the decades and centuries to scratch the surface on and say they figured it out. If you're not a woman, you haven't figured anything out.

It's partially due to the fact that as humans and as society has gone on we have evolved past the point that we no longer listen to our natural impulses, our gut feelings and the things that helped our ancestor survive for centuries.

Many times our partners will tell us were being ridiculous or irrational or overreacting. Sometimes they are trying to be reasonable and the calm one, other times its gaslighting.

They're not us, they're not inside our
head, or our body. And they didn't just
physically give birth to another life.

Having a baby will really put a relationship to
the test. How strong is your trust in your partner
that they will actually protect you, and take
care of you, and deny the whims of others.
That includes their mama.

Now let's start at the beginning.
6 in 10 marriages the wife does not get along
with the mother in law, and/or they kinda
get along with the father in law. Sometimes
its neither parent in law, and its strained.

When you're pregnant this can cause a lot of
unnecessary tension, your partner might feel
that they need to choose a side or play referee.

One thing that made a couple things towards
the end of the pregnancy very strained was in
my family and in my culture only a handful
of women that are part of your inner circle
may know the name of the baby before it's
born, or one of the names you have chosen.

They had a hard time with that, it wasn't
something they were used to, anything other than

what they knew or experienced growing up was different and a little hard to get your head around, but the grandparents respected us regardless and had questions. Which we welcomed.

Having a separate culture from your partners family can create strain and my husband is part of my culture and he chose it before we met, because his ancestors came from the same culture, and he wanted to keep tradition alive.

Some couples will experience pressure
and strain postnatal with some
parents, or even grandparents.
On either side of your family can argue a
ridiculous notion called "grandparents rights".

Let me make it very clear grandparents have no rights other than the rights you give them.

A woman postnatal goes through this
thing I call the mama bear reaction.

People will, right after you have a baby
start with this, "oh I want to hold the
baby. I want to see the baby."

Your in-laws or friends even Your family will try to bombard you in the hospital room and when you go home, the minute you are home.

You don't have to let anyone in, if you don't want to, it is not unreasonable to ask people to wait and not come over. Or not come to the hospital until after the baby has had its first doctors visit check up, and you've had time to adjust, heal, and bond and your spouse has had time to do the same.

I was very wary in the beginning about people holding my child, and that came from the mama bear response.
It's not in your head, you just gave birth to your offsprings and its your natural primal responses to protect that child. If you have a strained relationship or not good relationship with your mother-in-law or your mother or any member of either side of the families, you do not have to let them hold your baby, you can say no. If your spouse has a problem with it, tough taters. They're supposed to be supporting you and advocating for your choices.

Buy your spouse the books that are for the non pregnant person in the relationship so they know what they're supposed to do how they're supposed act if they don't know already.

A list of baby names are really important.
In my culture we believe a baby will
tell you their name and it'll be known

to you when they're born. When you
look upon the baby it will be clear.
So having a few suggestions is a good idea

You do not have to name your child,
the third, the Junior, the whatever…
just because it's a family tradition.

Its can actually be a big pain in the butt
for the child later in life, when the child
gets older and wants to establish their own
life and identity apart from its family.

We chose names that had personal meaning
to us that were sort of family names but
not family names we even use names
from some of our favorite fandoms.

Some of my friends that were pregnant
around the same time I was used names
that were not just from a fandom but pop-
culture. Because that's the way the times.

But what's most important, is to remember that
what sounds cute to you when you're pregnant
now, is the name they have to grow up with.
If you don't develop that connection to let
the baby commune with you and let you

know what they want, then chose wisely,
because playground bullies still exist.

And like me you do not have to tell
people what name you decided on.
You do not have to make a big post on
social media declaring you had a baby.
If people are upset with you because you didn't
post it online or personally told them that you
had a baby they're more or less following you
for the drama and Not because they care.

Sometimes people take advantage of the
fact that you are forgetful when you're
pregnant and expect you to keep promises
you made when you were pregnant. *"You
promised I could be a godmother"*

*"You promised father Patrick whatever or
reverend whatever could baptize the baby"*

You actually didn't promise anything you
probably said *"okay"* with the questioning
look like *(if I just agree now will you shut up
and leave me alone and stop pressuring me.)*

You don't owe anyone anything
when it comes to your child.

You have the right to withdraw
consent at anytime.

Sometimes people say pregnant women are
paranoid. Not actually true, for some very strange
reason when you're pregnant your perception can
be a little off, but your woman's intuition is not.

Ask someone you trust what things might
actually seem like, as opposed to maybe
confronting someone straight out, right away.

Pregnant women tend to worry more, especially
when they have had a traumatic birth experience
the first time, every movement, every kick,
every pain you worry something is wrong, and
something is going to be wrong this time.

I think if I called the doctors office nurse
once from the middle to the end of this
pregnancy, I called her like 20 times.

And sometimes once a week.

Postpartum PTSD

This is a little different than postpartum depression. Postpartum depression is a very serious thing and it needs to be addressed the moment someone notices it and immediately.

Postpartum PTSD is just what it sounds like.

PTSD is not limited to war and soldiers.

When I was pregnant with my first child there was no available healthcare, even though I fit the criteria for high-risk they did not accept my insurance, many of the doctors within a 10 mile radius did not accept my insurance or were accepting new patients either. So I had to see a midwife.

Because otherwise I would've had
to deliver the baby myself.
Because I chose to see a midwife as
my last resort option it made a lot
of things stressful at the time.
So I had to continue with the midwife
and the option for home birth because
there was a regular fear of what would
happen to me if I gave birth in hospital.

As time went on and I got closer to my due date, at my last ultrasound I had at 39 weeks, said that the baby was 6 pounds but 22 inches long. Well they read that wrong, they also missed a bone deformity that I had that would've made vaginal delivery impossible without severe danger to the child and myself. And the reason they missed is because the available medical services at the time and the location we're not experienced in seeing the condition. Because it is common in women of eastern European descent and the area I lived at the time that was primarily women of Latino descent. So they had no clue to look for it or even alert my midwife that there might be a complication. If anything they withheld my records altogether because they didn't directly work with this midwife so they felt they didn't have to tell her anything.

Fast forward to delivery when I went in to labor I was in a lot of pain all the techniques I learned didn't help me and I temporarily lost my vision from the pain, I was in so much pain the baby, was so big when he was finally born, and the struggle he and I had was so severe that caused him to have a Traumatic Brain Injury which he survived from. But my placenta wouldn't come out and

it was stuck they had to call an ambulance for
him and they had to call ambulance for me.
When we arrived at the hospital separately
the maternity ward staff and the labor and
delivery staff at the local hospital were cold,
rude, and impatient and they treated me
like an animal. They did not treat me like
a human, they we're almost abusive.

Because I had to go the route I did
with delivery and prenatal care,
I was not allowed to see my
baby for almost 24 hours.
I had to be evaluated by a mental health
professional, which was not necessary. I was
spoken to by physicians (I would've never seen
1 million years) like I was a complete moron.
And the nurses on the maternity floor had
the most dismissive attitude about the whole
situation they kept pushing medication on me
that I said *"No, I don't want to take this, because
I don't know what it is and I probably don't need
it."* And they said *"Well it's protocol."* I said *"I
don't care if it's protocol I don't know what it is."*

Finally my father intervened and called the
director of the hospital and our attorney and
things were handled a lot differently from there.
At least in the adult side of the hospital. I was
spoken to very rudely by the neonatal doctors.

I was told by the Neonatologists that everything
that happened was 100% my fault, and they
don't know what the outcomes going to be.
They need me to sign a DNR, they started
coming at me with all this extra stuff. I was just
allowed to see my child for the first time after
he was born because I never saw him when
he came out. Because of the vision loss, that's
where the term blackout pain comes from.

So between the staff treating me badly, the
whole experience of the birth and then these
Neonatal doctors telling me that I'm this
monster because, I had a difficult birth with my
child. It just compounded to the point where
my mother was by my side the entire time.
She said "I'm not leaving you alone with these
people." and she told the head of nicu "you
do not speak to her unless I or the attorneys
present, since many of your doctors can not do
so in a compassionate or civilized manner."

But the neonatal nurse were the best, we
had a couple nurses we didn't like,

But we have some we still talk to to this day.

This whole experience created the PTSD
for me from the birth experience.

That's why I was terrified the second time
around to have another child and that is why
my children were almost 8 years apart and I'm
glad I had my second child where I did because
between myself, my spouse and my second set
of doctors, and the children's hospital. we made
darn sure nothing like that happened again.

There are many really great doctors and
therapists that will work with women
who developed postpartum PTSD.
I'll include a listing on how to find
them in the appendix of the book

CHAPTER 7

THE QUIRKY ANECDOTES THAT SPARKED THE IDEA, TO WRITE A BOOK

And here is that humor I promised you in the beginning. If you hadn't noticed the cyanide sweet sarcasm that comes with your multiple weeks of pregnancy.
Then here is the humor.

The silly stuff, the stuff I wrote in the moments of embarrassment, and the moments of my friends embarrassment.

That comes with being pregnant.

Bumpism number 1

When you first start to getting bumpy, and your boobs bust out at the same time, you will almost suffocate putting your socks on.

Bumpism number 2

You fart under the blanket and pregnancy brain gives you a momentary laps of it happening and you pick up your blanket and shake it to bring it up over your shoulders,
Just to be hit with a fart smell. Congratulation you just Dutch ovened yourself!

Bumpism number 3

They lied to us about the subsequent pregnancies after the first being easier.

Bumpism number 4

When you have gestational diabetes,
And you have a lower than safe blood sugar,
And you have to narf half your stash of Girl Scout cookies to be able to bring it back up,
The Sugar Squrts are sure to follow. More on this to come.

Bumpism number 5

Multitasking!
When you are constantly needing the restroom but
trying to complete you handmade craft,
Get a small purse, and take it with you!
Wash your hands before you resume your project!

Bumpism number 6

When you buy maternity clothes in your pre pregnancy size and they are too big, thanks to first
trimester crash dieting.

Bumpism number 7

If you know your body, and yourself well enough
you can scare the resident doctors easily with big
words because after all, they are still students and
don't know as much as they think they do.

Bumpism number 8

It's no longer called vaginal discharge
Or vaginal mucus .....
It's called Pussy Boogers!

Bumpism number 9

When the second trimester comes and suddenly you are hungry again, except it's like the hunger of 4 teenage boys that smoked their first joint and now they have the munchies!

Bumpism number 10

Learn to scope out all routes and distance to all restrooms, so you have an exact plan of action, when duty calls 7 times in one dinner date night

Bumpism number 11

Things that may not bother you when you are not pregnant, but suddenly bother you when you are pregnant, you can develop a life long intolerance too. And then when pregnant again the reaction is amplified. Damn you raw onions.

Bumpism number 12

When hiking on a beginners trail, and you suddenly blitz to the closest outhouse,
Because even though breakfast was awesome, and you didn't puke, your body still says No.

You have now answered the age old question….. "Does a bear shit in the woods ?"

Yes Virginia, a bear shits in the wood and so does the pregnant lady!

Bumpism number 13

Just because you have GD doesn't mean your life is now salad, chicken, and rice till the fetus comes out. There are many excellent options for food that are not bland and limited.

Bumpism number 14

When you have previously bumped before the second bumping happens faster, and sometimes not as comfortably as the first time!

Bumpism number 15

When you are short and you realize your maternity pants come up under you boobs,
You just solved two major problems Comfortable pants + Boob sweat catcher = goals accomplished!

Bumpism number 16

If anyone has been wondering how the second trimester has been going, I just now found an M&M that I lost in my bra two days ago -SD

Bumpism number 17

When you are in the second trimester and you are no longer nauseous, but you don't have a Viking appetite, it must be a girl.

Bumpism number 18

When you hit the point in your pregnancy that you are just a little too big for pre pregnancy clothes and underwear and it's time to buy the specialty stuff. Your wallet will be crying.

Bumpism number 19

When your favorite holiday shirt fit during the first trimester but in the second trimester it's too snug… crying is ok.

Bumpism 20

When you finally find out all the puking during the first trimester added up to the gender you hoped for.

It makes all the nights of hugging the toilet, pulling over on the freeway, having a cop pull up behind you to ask if you need assistance... worth it.

Bumpism Number 21

There is this rare undeclared symptom, Diaflaticonstaitis

Essentially the slow digestive tract creates pockets of air = Flatulence

That blocks stool from passing without out struggling = Constipation

And from your body being irritated it activates the emergency evacuation system and makes the dumping process happen = Diarrhea

If it wasn't blocked by a pocket of air = Flatulence

And when that nuke, that's been marinating since the start of the week hits, you anger an old injury from bracing yourself during the surge, causing a flair up of pain = Arthritis

And that Boys and Girls is part of the miracle of pregnancy.

Bumpism number 22

The book says after week 16 the breast pain stops I call bullshit.

Bumpism number 23

Just because it was your favorite vegetable before pregnancy doesn't mean your body is in love with it now.

Bumpism number 24

According to my husband- The reasons you pee yourself when you sneeze after you just peed is because... when you first peed you only emptied your primary bladder, your secondary bladder fills during pregnancy, reserving urine just for when you're about to sneeze. Regardless of the time you emptied the primary bladder.

The way he delivered this nugget of dude knowledge made it sound almost scientifically sound even though it's not.

Bumpism number 25

When your pain is caused by Relaxin

(I know a man invented this word)

And suddenly all the hip bones and pelvic bones start to really shift, it's like Mother Nature is hoofing you in the front butt.

And it's not like the first pregnancy it's stronger because you have nerve damage from the first natural birth!

Bumpism number 26

Nothing like having a sprained dominant foot while pregnant

Now I can waddle and limp.

Bumpism Number 27

You have hit a certain point in your bump growth that your favorite bath towel no longer wraps around you.

Bumpism Number 28

When you walk into your local Target and there are 9 other women all looking just as pregnant as you are and your husband exclaimed "looks like no one else practiced social distancing either…"

Bumpism number 29

You find new uses for big cleaning appliances

Like … who needs a broom, when you have a shop vac. Or why bother with a mop, when you have a rug scrubber, it does hard floors too.

Bumpism number 30

Spaghetti and meatballs might sound good but it might turn you inTo a vomit breathing dragon as well.

And only, a left over baby shower cupcake is going to save you!

Bumpism 31

Pregnancy and summer heat

No. Just no.

Bumpism number 32

Most of the pregnancy pants out there do not compensate for summer heat and just add layers to your already hot and overheated belly

I have found cotton pettie pants and a dress are a great alternative for those among us with no thigh gap, and cotton bike shorts help too.

Bumpism number 33

Did you ever wonder why men have a dip in their waist when they side sleep?

It's so you can prop your pregnancy leg up on it, to give yourself proper pelvic pain relief and to elevate those kankles!!!

Bumpism Number 34

There are hundreds of "miracle belly creams", but nothing works like Vicks cream in the summer.

Bumpism Number 35

You don't realize how many muscles you use to laugh with until you give birth. Then suddenly you go from *"don't make me pee.", to "don't make me bust my kitty stitches."*

Bumpism Number 36

When you feel like you are 14.5 months pregnant suddenly you are tougher than the most harden criminal.

Because you are big, and overwhelmed, and over heated, and just over it!

Bumpism Number 37

When you drop something, and it disappears into the void that is under your bump and boobs.

Don't worry it's only temporary!

Bumpism number 38

They lie to you about all the discomfort of a second pregnancy.

Example any pain you didn't have with the first you will have mostly likely experience with the second.

And the doctors responded to this question with "because you've already stretched once before, you'll stretch faster and further the second time."

Bumpism Number 39

Any eloquence you might have had is gone. When you are so far along, you end up saying things that clearly needed more elaboration like "I have never eaten five guys nuts!" when you should have said "I have never had a chance to try the complementary peanuts at five guys".

Bumpism Number 40

When you go to a restaurant and the server sits you at a booth and you say, "sorry this won't work I am way too pregnant to fit in a space that small"

And the child server reply's "Oh, I couldn't tell" WTF does that mean.

Did he just call me fat? Its on like donkey kong.

Bumpism number 41

When you want to do something sexy for your partner and you realize all your sexy lingerie is from before pregnancy Sexy outfits become a few scarves and in my case a cold unopened craft beer between your boobs.

Bumpism number 42

I don't know about your hometowns, but every time I am really craving something awesome

Or simple

The place is out of stock. Or they messed up your order so badly you burst into tears and rage.

You think these people would understand "you don't cross or piss off a pregnant woman."

Bumpism number 43

Between the pelvic floor pain, fibromyalgia, the kankles, the gastritis, the heartburn, the loss of feeling in your fingers or constant relocating them. It's amazing that we do this multiple times.

Apparently your brain releases an automatic restart chemical that makes you forget everything you suffered. I call BS.

Bumpism Number 44

If this isn't your second or greater full term pregnancy then you might not be familiar with the neuropathy pain you acquired with a previous birth

Now granted if you gave birth vaginally you are familiar with something called "the ring of fire" it's that intense burning you feel in your labia as the baby starts to crown

Now it's pregnancy number 2 and you are experiencing the nerve damage pain from the first pregnancy even if you are still 6 weeks from your due date.

A cool bead compress works great for this.

Bumpism number 46

Crying over a food not being available when ordering is not irrational. It's a hair trigger response and unless someone is pregnant they just don't understand.

Bumpism Number 47

Alkaline heartburn

Better known as gastric napalm.

It can start at random and anything will trigger it, nothing gets rid of it.

But the baby will have a lot of hair because of it.

Bumpism number 48

I now know why villains rub their hands together when they say Mwahaha

It's because they have 3rd trimester carpal tunnel syndrome too.

Bumpism Number 49

You'll be running to the hospital with a false alarms in these last few weeks of pregnancy probably two times before you actually go into labor.

Bumpism Number 50

Now I know why Dracula was always portrayed in the old films laying on his back with his arms crossed over his chest it's not because he wasn't practicing being dead it's because he had pregnancy carpal tunnel too.

Now I've mentioned the carpal tunnel twice that's not because it's funny,. but it's because it's the other hand and joint symptom that can happen during the 3rd trimester That doesn't always happen with your first baby but can happen with sub sequential pregnancies. You can also get loosening of your finger joints to where dislocating and relocating your finger is a common every day occurrence.

Bumpism number 51

Pregnancy brain

It's something you don't think about or remember from your first pregnancy but you suddenly have a state of brain farts and when you were supposed to be cooking dinner you made dessert instead.

I hope you had a good giggle with that and it had some relatable moments.

THE APPENDIX

THE LEXICON OF ACRONYMS

HEG Hyperemesis gravidarum

A condition in which you develop either early or late in pregnancy that includes extreme vomiting without the ability to keep anything down with the chance of dehydration.

GD Gestational Diabetes

IBS D

Irritable bowel syndrome with diarrhea

PCOS

Poly cystic ovarian syndrome

IgA deficiency

Immunoglobulin A deficiency

Is common in Scandinavian people and
results in the antibodies and immunoglobulin
response in your mucous membranes to be
weaker than other people. It is genetic but
you can't pass it to someone like an STD.
Either they get the genes for it or they don't.

NICU
Neonatal ICU

UTI
Urinary Track Infection.

HELLP Syndrom

HELLP syndrome is a pregnancy complication that
affects the blood and liver. It's a medical emergency
that needs quick treatment. Signs and symptoms of
HELLP include blurry vision, chest pain or pain in
the upper right or middle part of the belly, swelling
and throwing up.

Bumpism

A pop-culture reference created by the author to explain the experience and diversity of pregnancy.

Books referenced

What to expect when expecting
1973 copy of Merck Manual
Justin wilson: homegrown Louisiana cookin'

Culture references

Aboriginal child birthing techniques, out of print book and or spoken oral traditions.

Clothing

walmart.com
torrid.com
Kindredbravely.com
thediaryfairy.com
carolwrightgifts.com
romans.com

Postpartum psychology

pyschologytody.com
Search postpartum.

Breat Pumps

aeroflowbreastpumps.com
www.medela.us

Birth Plans

Basically go to google and type
in birth plan templet.
I also used the birth plan templet
from Kindred Bravely.

Notes:

Notes:

Notes:

Notes:

Notes:

CHAPTER 8

THE CHAPTER I HOPE YOU DON'T NEED. BUT IF YOU DO, I WILL BE HERE

Sometimes birth goes well, baby comes out everything went according to plan, the pregnancy was fine.

But then sometimes…
You have an experience like I did. That you just read about in pregnancy psychology.

Baby comes out and there is something wrong. It might be something like the cleft lip and palate or just the palate, that is fixable it comes with it's challenges, but it is fixable and it's a bit of a stay in the NICU which is the neo-natal intensive care unit.

Sometimes you have things happen like my friend
did, Where the cord may have been wrapped
around the babies throat or you have a struggle
like I did, and your baby suffers a traumatic brain
injury and you have lifelong struggles But that
baby doesn't give up fighting, and neither do you.

Sometimes you have a second pregnancy
like I did, and You have the preeclampsia
and your baby was born early.

Your baby is born even three weeks early,
But when they come out and you don't
hear a cry and you wait, and wait … when
you hear the cry and it's the best thing
you have heard in the entire world. You
breathe out that breath you were holding.

But then they say "emergency" and we have
to trying get the babies heart rate up.
Because gestational diabetes, can cause
heart defects in unborn babies that are
completely undetectable until they're born
because, the heart beats differently in the
womb than it does outside of the womb.

It is all very scary and your baby will not be
in the maternity nursery, the baby will not
be in the room with you like you planned.

The baby might be down the hall in or on another
floor in the Neo Natal intensive care unit.

With my first child he was only a few floors
down. With my second child they were in
the children's hospital across the road.
My husband did a lot of walking.
Which he gladly did.

I had to pump breast milk both times,
Neither baby was able to latch on.

The hard part came when I got to go to the NICU
both times and I couldn't stay the whole time.

The first time the baby was in ward
like setting, that had a bunch of
incubators or isolettes in one room.

The first time I didn't know what was going
on. I felt alone because I was the only mom in
there with a full term baby. Until about three
weeks passed and I was eating my dinner and
there was another mom that spoke to me,
asking me if i was ok? Or did I need hot sauce!
Because she had a stash.

And I'm going use a pseudonym for
her, the nickname that we called her

by, it was her nickname she had her
whole life but her name was Pig.
And she later had introduced me
to Cat. She helped me
Stand up and not take the crap
attitudes from people.

The second time around. This children's hospital
had it set up that everyone had an individual
room. I could stay as long as I wanted, I could
stay overnight, and I chose to stay by bedside
the entire time as long as I could. I did take days
where I went home and my husband stayed.

And it made for a great experience
because it made pumping easier.

But I was also the veteran mom on the floor. As
hard as it was being a NICU mom twice, in a
way I was that beacon of hope for the parents
that were there for the first time. That had
never seen the inside of a place like this and
didn't know what was going on or happening.

When I would run into them in the hallways,
or in the family lunchroom, having breakfast,
lunch, dinner, just taking a break, or they were
coming in for the first time I would introduce

myself and ask them "Is this your first time
here?" and I would keep my tone comforting
but jovial to distract them from their fear.
And it was more often that it was one of the dads,
and they would say "yes. yes, they told me to go
wait in here, I don't know what's happening."

And I would tell them it's okay, they have to
take report, get everything set up, get the baby
set up, do all the vitals, make sure everything is
ready. It going to be some long nights in a place
that's not home. And it might not have been what
you thought would happen, when you and your
spouse planned it out. But it can only get better.
And they would feel better, and ask me "Is
this your first baby?", and I would respond
"No, this is my second NICU baby."

And then when their wives would come over,
and they are able to see their babies, If I
was in the hall or I going to the ice machine
(they had the good ice) or coming back from
eating after pumping, they would stop me and
say "hey this is a lady, I told you about."
And the moms would hug me. And they
would say "thank you for you reaching
out." and I would tell them if you see me
and need to talk or cry. I am here.

So it gave them someone that they could relate
with and share a similar experience with.

The hardest part for me was going
home, Without my baby.

We have a big rocking chair in our living
room and I sat in that rocking chair a lot
of my pregnancy, I rocked back and forth
while watching Gordon Ramsay yell at
people, which was very relaxing for me.

And I dreamed about being able to bring
my baby home, Rock them in that chair,
feed them during late nights. But that
didn't go according to plan right away.

Some stays in the neonatal intensive care unit can
be months, but sometimes it's weeks. with my
first child it was two days short of two months.

And because of my parents and the
friends I made at the hospital, the other
moms made the time go by faster and
made all the difference in the world.

For the second time it was only a
few weeks and it seemed like a long
time but it went by very quickly.

And sometimes… We come home empty.

Instead of planning for the two week meet
the baby. We are planning a funeral.
Stillbirths happen, unfortunate
accidents during delivery happen.
Sometimes the husband comes home
with the Baby, but you don't. That's not
your fault and it's not his either.

It's a reality of childbirth that few
doctors today take seriously.
They worry about their career and their
high numbers. Not your life or that baby's
and they take risks they should not.

It takes a long time to heal from this pain.

It takes a long time to find your center again.

Having a miscarriage, having a stillbirth,
is not a result of a Lack Of Faith. And
don't let anyone tell you differently.

Things just happen. Miscarriages happen,
preterm labor happens for a million different
reasons. Some with early intervention are
preventable. But not 100%, and not every time.

Stillbirths can present suddenly and you
have no way of knowing or planning how
you're going to handle the outcome.

Some babies are born disabled. And you make
a choice how you want to handle that.

I hope you never have to read this chapter.
I hope you never have to feel as a spouse,
the helplessness of watching your partner
suffer in watching And waiting to find out
the outcome of the survival of your child.

I hope as mother your time sitting by an
Isolette or incubator is short and you get
to go home with your baby quickly.

And I hope you never go through the pain of
loss that comes with losing a child to soon.

Like I said at chapter title.

I hope you never need this chapter, I
hope you never have to read it.
I'm here if you need me, and if you
need me, you will know.